Mediterranean Diet Recipes

The Complete Guide with Easy-To-Make, Quick, And Flavorful Everyday Recipes to Lose Weight and Improve Your Health

Jennifer Benson

Table of Contents

damages that may befall them after undertaking information described herein.

Additionally, the information in the following page is intended only for information purposes and should thus be thought of as universal. As befitting its nature, it is presented without assurance regarding its prolonged validity or interim quality. Trademarks that are mentioned are done without written consent and can be in no way be considered an endorsement from the trademark holder.

Mediterranean Sea Diet

Over view

The Mediterranean Sea diet is per harps the healthiest diet one can rely on. It implies a common dietary pattern which, for ages has been practiced by the people living in the Mediterranean countries. The different cultures within the basin contributed to the emergence of various natural plants as the main source of food, typically olive tree, wheat, grapevine, orange, lemon trees, tomatoes, eggplants, corn, rice, potatoes, asparagus, mangoes and among others. Moreover, the adverse effects of the artificially manufactured foods, red meat, and fatty foods have been highly discouraged in the Mediterranean diet. Besides, the fruits and natural whole foods, the Mediterranean diet is rich with various herbs such as kale, parmesan, parsley, basil, rosemary, cinnamon, sage, pepper, mint, and nutmeg; that are significant in treating and overcoming the development of severe illness in human being.

However, it is significant to note that the Mediterranean diet stands out distinctively among other diets that contain a high percentage of calorie, fat, sugar, and artificially added ingredients. Above and beyond, vegetables such as garlic, chili, onions, tomatoes among others make Mediterranean diet so flavorful and tasty. It is such taste and natural deliciousness and sweetness that has spanned the consumption of Mediterranean Sea diet foods. The Mediterranean

Sea diet takes various forms of preparation; it can be prepared as a salad with variety of vegetables, leaves, fruits, and herbs, the fruits can be used for making naturally sweet juice and smoothies, the grains, corn, potatoes, and rice can be used to prepare healthy whole foods to boost one's energy levels. Seeds also feature commonly in Mediterranean Sea diet such as sunflower seeds, pumpkin seeds, sesame seeds, among others.

Mediterranean Sea recipes

There are several Mediterranean Sea recipes that you can choose from depending on your choice and preference. It ranges from vegetable and green food recipes to seafood and whole grain recipes. However, it is imperative to note that all the Mediterranean recipes have health benefits making it the best diet for anyone to enjoy to improve on their health.

Fruit Mediterranean Sea Diet Recipe

Undoubtedly, fruits are the omega and an outstanding source of vitamins, which are important in building the human body immune system. They are also an important source of antioxidant that cleanses the body. The recipes include;

Pear and ginger pudding

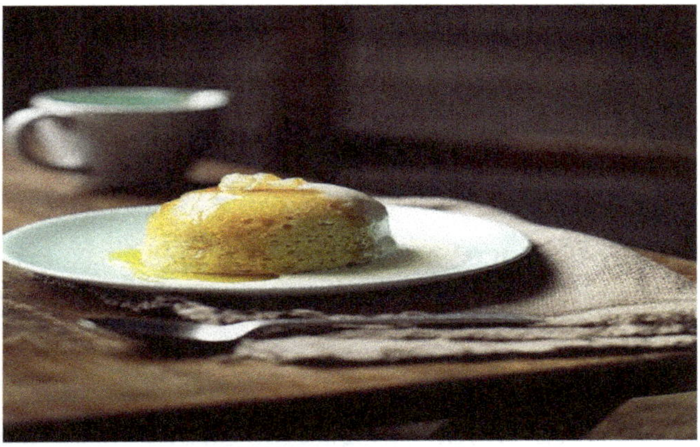

Ingredients

- 1 ripe pear
- Golden syrup
- 1 large free-range egg
- 55g of self-raising flour
- 1 piece of stem ginger in syrup
- 55g of unsalted butter
- 55g of caster sugar
- 1 orange

Directions

- Place 2 teacups upside down on greaseproof paper, draw round them.
- Cut out the circles.

- Grease one side with butter, then grease the inside of the teacups.
- Using a food processor, process the flour together with the sugar, butter, and egg.
- Add the ginger, orange zest, pulse twice.
- Pour a small golden syrup into the base of each cup, top with half the chopped pear each.
- Divide the batter between the two cups, then lightly press a circle of paper on top, butter-side down.
- Let cook in the microwave, full power for 4 minutes.
- Let cool.
- Serve and enjoy with lashings of hot custard.

Berry good pancakes

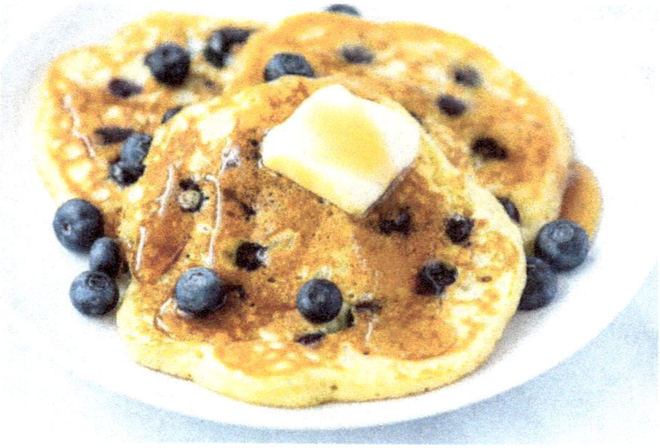

Ingredients

- 1 handful of blueberries
- 1 cup self-rising flour

- 6 slices of streaky bacon
- 1 teaspoon baking powder
- 1 large free-range egg
- 20g of butter
- 1 cup of milk

Directions

- Crack the eggs, fill the same cup with flour.
- Add to the bowl. Toss in the baking powder.
- Fill the cup with milk, add a tiny pinch of sea salt.
- Whisk till smooth. Cover the bowl in Clingfilm and put to one side.
- Heat a non-stick frying pan, let fry until crisp.
- Put a large frying pan on a medium heat, melt the butter.
- Place the pancake batter into the pan.
- Let cook 2 minutes, until little bubbles rise up to the top. Turnover.
- Dot a handful of blueberries across the half-cooked pancakes.
- Transfer to a plate and cover with foil.
- Add the remaining butter, use all the butter.
- Serve and enjoy with the bacon.

Cranberry granola

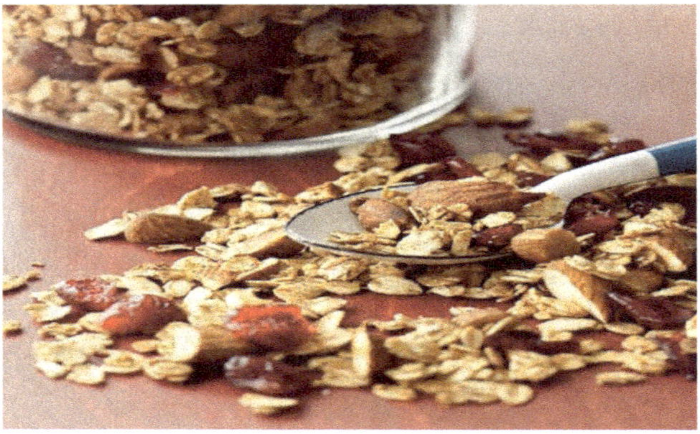

Ingredients

- 2 tablespoons of vegetable oil
- Runny honey
- 400g of jumbo rolled oats
- 100g of seeds
- 200g of mixed nuts
- 150g of dried cranberries
- 1 teaspoon of ground cinnamon
- 500g of plain yoghurt

Directions

- Begin by preheating your oven ready to 350°F.
- Mix the nuts with the oats, half the cranberries, seeds, and the oil. Stir.
- Divide between 2 baking sheets, let cook for 25 minutes till golden.
- Mix the yoghurt together with the cinnamon.

- Serve the granola with the yoghurt and a drizzle of honey.
- Enjoy.

Passion fruit cairipinha

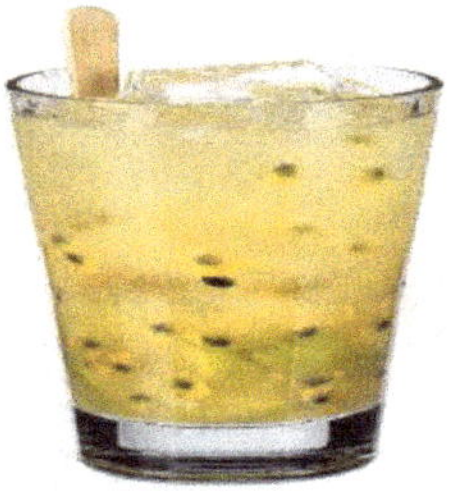

Ingredients

- 4 tablespoons of golden caster sugar
- Crushed ice
- 3 limes
- 75ml of cachaça
- 1 ripe passion fruit

Directions

- Begin by cutting the limes into wedges.
- Place the lime wedges except 2 with sugar in a cocktail shaker.
- Muddle briefly to almost dissolve the sugar.
- Add the cachaça, spoon in most of the passion fruit pulp.
- Fill the shaker with crushed ice and shake for 1 minute.

- Pour the cocktail into 2 glasses.
- Use the 2 remaining lime wedges to garnish and the passion fruit pulp.
- Serve and enjoy.

Apple and cranberry sauce

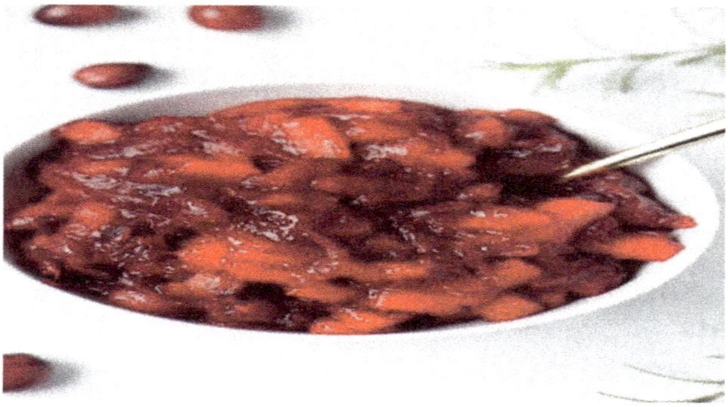

Ingredients

- 1 stick of cinnamon
- 500g of cranberries
- 150g of golden caster sugar
- 2 bramley apples

Directions

- Place all the ingredients in a wide saucepan with a splash of water.
- Place the pan on heat and bring to the boil.
- Simmer gently until the cranberries have burst and the apple are soft.

- Boil down until the mixture thickens slightly.
- Remove, let cool.

Date, cocoa and pumpkin recipe

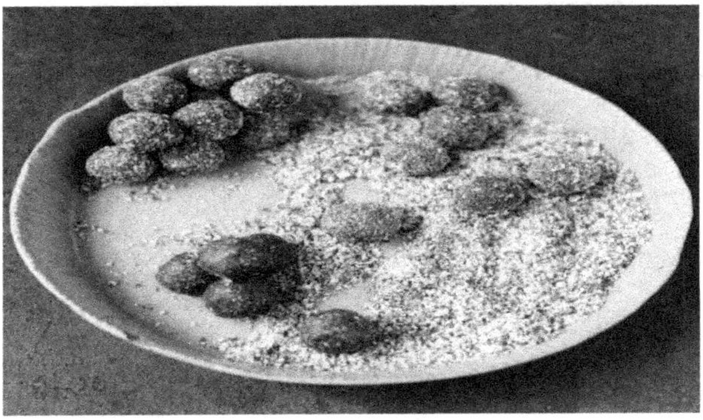

Ingredients

- 1 teaspoon of vanilla extract
- 1 orange
- 50g of whole almonds
- 80g of Medjool dates
- 1cm piece of fresh turmeric
- ½ teaspoon of ground cinnamon
- 20g of puffed brown rice
- 1 heaped teaspoon of quality cocoa powder
- 70g of pumpkin seeds
- ½ tablespoon of Manuka honey

Directions

- Expressly, blend 40g pumpkin seeds into a dust in a food processor.
- Add remaining pumpkin seeds with the puffed rice in the processor, almonds, and dates. Blend to chop.
- Add the ground turmeric, with cinnamon, cocoa powder, and a pinch of sea salt.
- Blend again until ground
- Add the vanilla together with the honey and half the orange juice.
- Blend briefly.
- Divide into 24 then roll into balls.
- Throw into the pumpkin seed dust.
- Shake to coat, storing them in the excess dust until needed.
- Serve and enjoy.

Cherry clafoutis

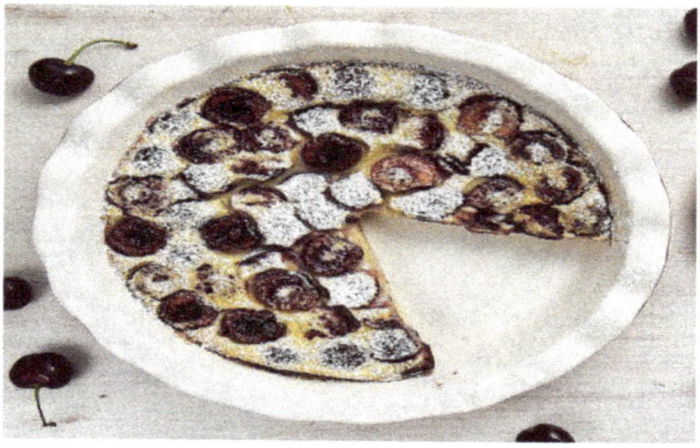

Ingredients

- 60g of sugar

- ½ tablespoon of unsalted butter
- 1 tablespoon of sugar
- ½ teaspoon of vanilla extract
- 300g of cherries
- 300ml of milk
- Icing sugar
- ½ teaspoon of baking powder
- 3 large free-range eggs
- 60g of plain flour

Directions

- Preheat the oven to 360°F.
- Combine plain four together with the baking powder, eggs, sugar, milk, and vanilla extract in a food processor, blend until smooth, keep for 30 minutes.
- Oil a round baking dish with the softened butter.
- Sprinkle over with the sugar.
- Dot the cherries around the base, place in the oven for 5 minutes.
- Remove and pour over the batter until the cherries are just covered.
- Return to the oven let bake for 35 minutes.
- Dust the clafoutis with icing sugar and serve warm.
- Enjoy.

Cranberry Bakewell

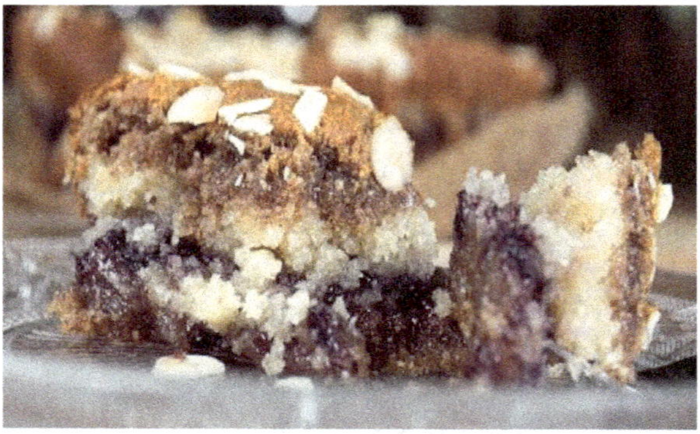

Ingredients

- 2 large eggs
- 375g of sweet short crust pastry
- 2 heaped tablespoons of plain flour
- 1 splash calvados
- 1 handful of cranberries, fresh, defrosted
- 250g of unsalted butter
- 1 orange
- 100g of icing sugar
- 375g of cranberries, fresh or defrosted
- 150g of golden caster sugar
- 1-star anise
- 1 orange
- 1/2 teaspoon of ground cinnamon
- 1 vanilla pod
- 300g of ground almonds
- 300g of golden caster sugar

Directions

- Grate the orange zest into a pan.
- Squeeze in the juice, let simmer with the remaining ingredients, stirring occasionally.
- Taste, and adjust accordingly.
- Cool, then remove the star anise.
- Roll out the pastry to line oiled loose-bottomed tart tin.
- Let chill in the fridge for 1 hour.
- Combine vanilla pod, almonds, plain flour, caster sugar, eggs, unsalted butter, and processor, process until smooth.
- Wrap in Clingfilm and chill in the fridge for 30 minutes with pastry.
- Preheat the oven ready to 380°F.
- Line the pastry with greaseproof paper and fill with dried beans.
- Let bake for 10 minutes.
- Remove the beans and paper continue to bake for more 15 minutes.
- Remove.
- Then, spread the pastry with the jam, dollop over the frangipane.
- Sprinkle with the cranberries, scatter with flaked almonds.
- Bake 55 minutes.
- Let tart cool.
- Grate the orange zest into a small bowl.

- Add the icing sugar, squeeze enough orange juice to give a drizzling consistency.
- Serve and enjoy with crème fraiche.

Winter ginger, pear and almond cake

The winter ginger, pear and almond recipe is known for its aromatic ginger flavor with spicy sweet satisfying ingredients. It is an incredible Mediterranean Sea fruit recipe for a perfect breakfast choice.

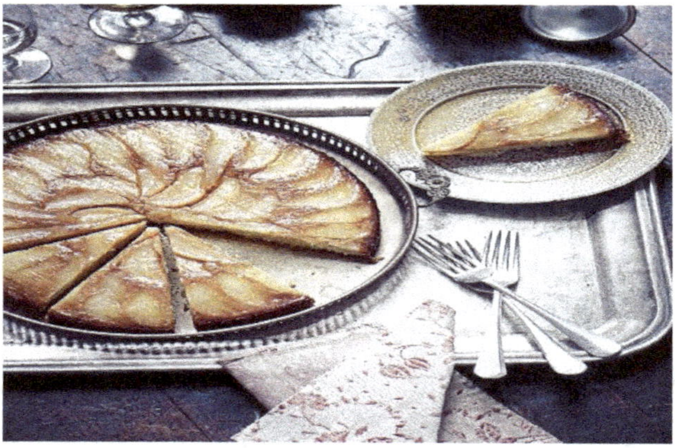

Ingredients

- 20g of butter
- 220g of ground almonds
- 300g of ginger
- 4 pears
- 200g of butter
- 1 vanilla pod

- 200g of caster sugar
- 550g of caster sugar
- 4 large free-range eggs

Directions

- Preheat the oven ready to 380°F.
- Place the vanilla pod, grated ginger, and pears into a pan.
- Add 400g sugar and water let boil, simmer for briefly.
- Lower the pears into the hot liquid, simmer for 10 minutes.
- Remove the pears from the liquid let cool.
- Line a cake tin with greaseproof paper.
- Combine the remaining 150g sugar and water in a pan over a high heat.
- Simmer for 15 minutes until dark golden brown.
- Stir in the butter until you get a caramel, then pour into cake tin.
- Slices cooled pears, arrange in the warm caramel.
- Mix butter with sugar until smooth.
- Add the eggs one at a time, mix well one after the other.
- Add the almonds and mix to combine.
- Pour the cake mixture over the pears let bake 35 minutes in the heated oven.
- Serve and enjoy.

Summer pudding

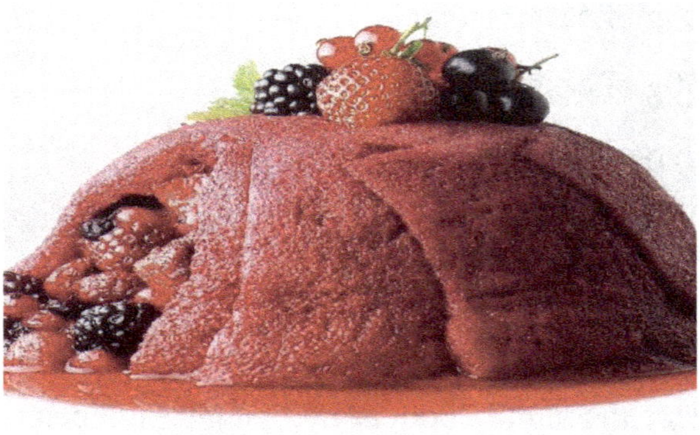

Ingredients

- 2 tablespoons of red berry jam
- 150g of sugar
- ½ of an orange
- ½ teaspoon of vanilla paste
- 800g of mixed summer berries
- Olive oil
- 7 large slices of white bread

Directions

- Grease a pudding basin with oil.
- Align with 2 sheets of Clingfilm.
- Place the berries in a large saucepan together with the sugar, orange juice, and vanilla paste.
- Over low heat, let cook for 5 minutes or till the juices start bleeding from the fruit. Let cool.
- Remove the crusts from the bread, spread over the jam.

- Line the basin with 6 of the slices, jam-side up with no gaps.
- Press the bread against the sides.
- Spoon the cooled fruit and pour its juice into the lined basin, reserving some.
- Cover the pudding with the last slice of bread, jam-side down.
- Place a saucer that fits inside the basin on top of the pudding, then place a weight, on top.
- Refrigerate 12 hours to soak the juices.
- Strain the leftover juice through a fine sieve into a small pan.
- Let boil, simmer for 10 minutes.
- Drizzle large slices with the syrup.
- Serve and enjoy with crème fraiche.

Raspberry burnt cream

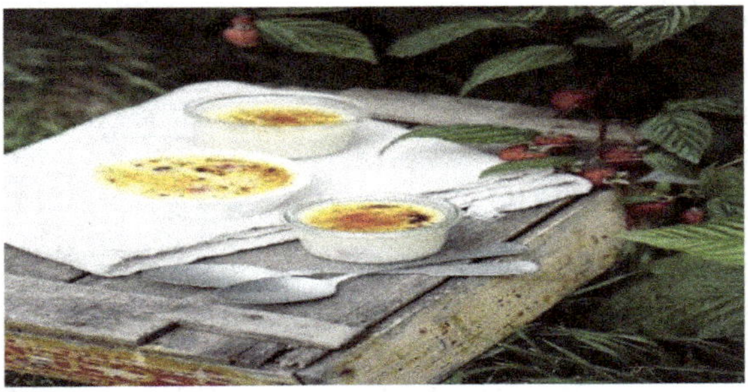

Ingredients

- 100g of raspberries
- 150ml of double cream
- 4 large free-range egg yolks

- 1 vanilla pod
- 2 tablespoons of golden caster sugar
- 150ml of single cream

Directions

- Preheat the oven to 300°F.
- Add vanilla pod to a pan with the creams over a low heat.
- In a bowl, whisk the egg yolks with sugar.
- Add in the hot cream, whisk frequently to make a custard.
- Strain through a sieve into a jug.
- Boil water.
- Divide the berries between four small ovenproof ramekins, then fill each with the custard.
- Place ramekins in roasting tray, pour in hot water halfway up the sides.
- Let cook in the oven for 20 minutes.
- Remove, let cool, then cover each ramekin with Clingfilm, refrigerate overnight.
- Sprinkle sugar over the custards, burn the top with a blowtorch.
- Allow to stand to let the burnt sugar hardens, then return to the fridge and chill until needed.
- Enjoy.

Citrus poached pears

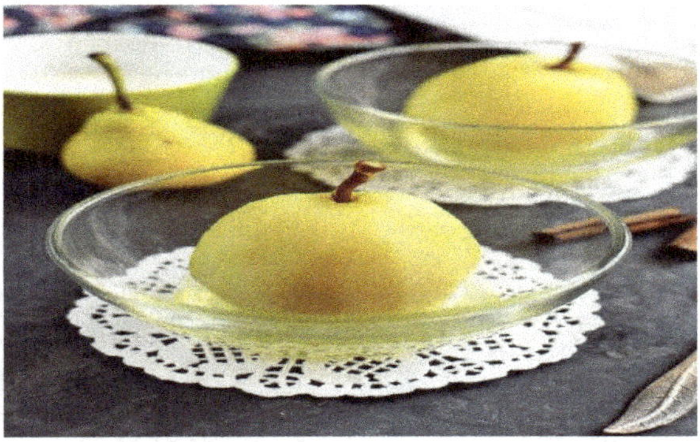

Ingredients

- Double cream
- 1 lemon
- 2 pears
- 1 stick of cinnamon
- 200g of granulated sugar
- 1 orange

Directions

- Place the peeled zest and juice from the lemon, orange into a saucepan.
- Add the cinnamon together with the sugar, add 500ml of water and bring to the boil, until the sugar dissolves.
- Add the pears into the syrup once the sugar has dissolved.
- Let simmer 12 minutes or until tender.
- Remove and let cool.
- Serve the pears with double cream and or with 4 tablespoons of poaching.

- Enjoy.

Limon cello and fruit salad fro-yo

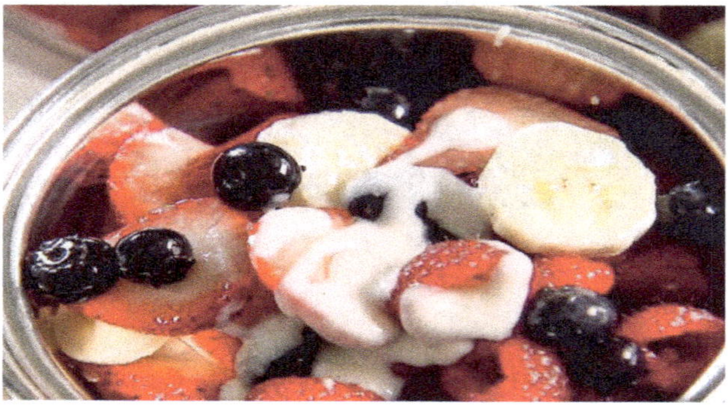

Ingredients

- 75ml of Limon cello
- 1kg of chopped mixed fruit
- Ice-cream cones
- 250ml of fat-free natural yoghurt
- Runny honey

Directions

- Blend the fruit together with the yoghurt, 2 tablespoons of honey, and the lemon cello in a food processor until smooth.
- Taste and adjust accordingly.
- Spoon into a dish and freeze for 2 hours, until frozen.
- Remove and place back into the processor, blend again to break up any ice crystals. Enjoy.

Vegetable Mediterranean recipes

Vegetables are the heart and a true definition of a Mediterranean Sea diet. It is the origin of all the health benefits associated with the Mediterranean Sea diet together with the fruits that make the Mediterranean meals complete.

Versatile veggie chili

The versatile veggie chili recipe is quite delicious and a hearty substitution to traditional chili. It features butternut squash, leek and spring onions for a greater flavor coupled with cayenne pepper for a perfect choice of a Mediterranean Sea diet.

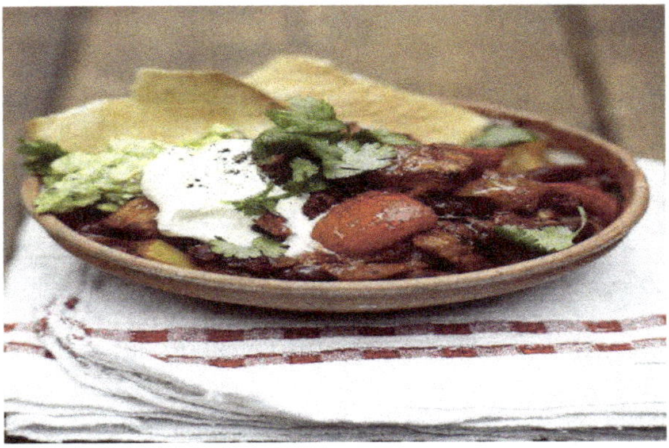

Ingredients

- 1 heaped teaspoon ground cumin
- Lime or lemon juice, or vinegar
- Olive oil
- 2 mixed-color peppers

- 2 cloves of garlic
- 1 level teaspoon cayenne pepper
- 2 x 400g of tins of beans
- 1 bunch of fresh coriander
- 2 fresh mixed-color chilies
- 1 onion
- 1 level teaspoon ground cinnamon
- 2 x 400g of tins of quality plum tomatoes
- 500g of sweet potatoes

Directions

- Preheat the oven ready to 400°F.
- Prepare and place chopped potatoes onto a baking tray.
- Sprinkle with a pinch of cayenne, cinnamon, cumin, sea salt and black pepper.
- Drizzle with oil then toss to coat.
- Let roast for 1 hour or until golden.
- Place 2 tablespoons of oil in a large pan over a medium-high heat.
- Add the onion together with peppers, and garlic.
- Let cook for 5 minutes, stirring regularly.
- Add the coriander stalks together with the chilies and spices.
- Cook for more 10 minutes or until softened, stirring occasionally.
- Add the beans, juice and all.

- Tip in the tomatoes, breaking them up with the back of a spoon, stir well.
- Let boil, lower the heat to medium-low for 30 minutes.
- Stir the roasted sweet potato through the chili with most of the coriander leaves,
- Taste and adjust accordingly.
- Add a squeeze of lime or lemon juice or a swig of vinegar.
- Serve and enjoy with yogurt or sour cream.

Classic ratatouille

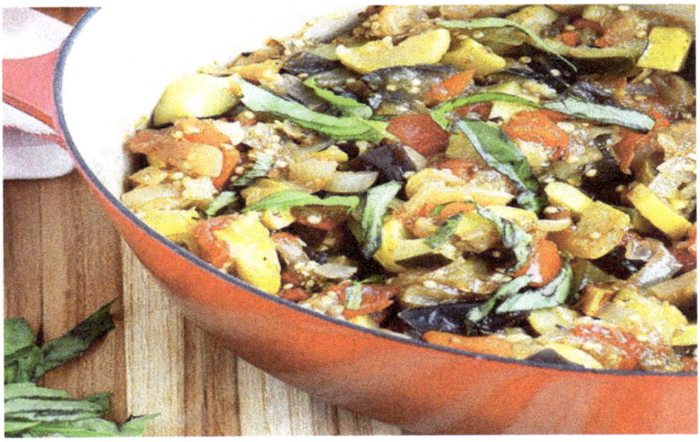

Ingredients

- 2 red onions
- 4 cloves of garlic
- 2 aborigines
- 3 courgettes
- 3 red or yellow peppers

- 6 ripe tomatoes
- ½ a bunch of fresh basil
- Olive oil
- A few sprigs of fresh thyme
- 1 x 400 g tin of quality plum tomatoes
- 1 tablespoon of balsamic vinegar
- ½ of a lemon

Directions

- Start by heating 2 tablespoons of oil in a large casserole pan over a medium heat.
- Add the chopped aubergines together with the courgettes and peppers.
- Let fry for 5 minutes, spoon the cooked vegetables into a large bowl.
- Add the onion, garlic, basil stalks, and thyme leaves with another drizzle of oil to the pan.
- Let fry for 15 minutes or until golden.
- Return the cooked veggie to the pan.
- Stir in the fresh and tinned tomatoes together with the balsamic and a pinch of sea salt and black pepper.
- Cover and let simmer over a low heat for 35 minutes.
- Tear in the basil leaves, grate in the lemon zest.
- Taste and adjust seasoning accordingly.
- Serve and enjoy with steamed rice.

Carrot spinach juice

Combining carrots with spinach provides a rich source of iron, calcium, and vitamins along with other mineral. It is a tastier Mediterranean juice with a simple step-by-step method.

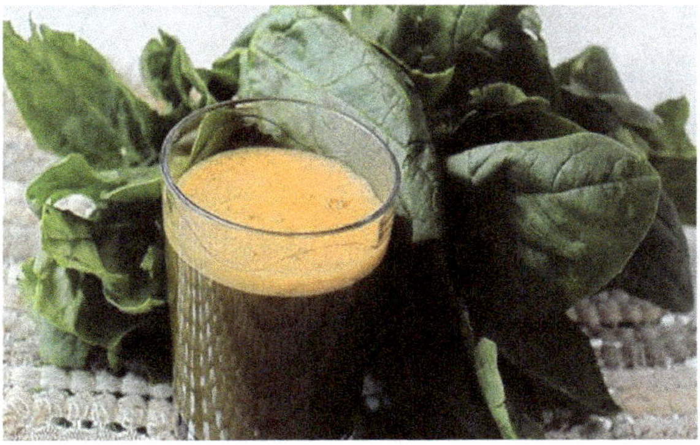

Ingredients

- 6 medium size carrots
- 1 large bunch of spinach
- Celery stalk
- ½ of lemon
- 1 ½ cups of water

Directions

- Combine the carrots together with the celery stalk and all the water in a blender.
- Blend to puree.
- Then, add the spinach and juice of lemon, (squeeze).

- Blend briefly, then, strain.
- Serve and enjoy.

Fresh tomato juice

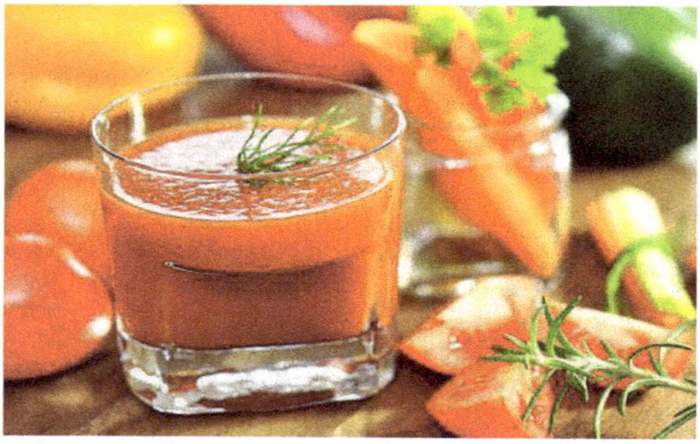

Ingredients

- Celery stalks
- Salt
- 2 ice cubes
- ¼ teaspoon of ground black pepper
- 2 carrots
- 6 ripe tomatoes

Directions

- Place tomatoes together with the carrots and celery in a blender.
- Blend until smooth.
- Then, add salt with black pepper to season, mix well.

- Add the ice cubes in serving glasses.
- Serve and enjoy.

Aubergine parmigiana

This a great meal recipe originating from the parts of northern Italy making a perfect Mediterranean Sea diet with variety of vegetables. It can be served perfectly with roasted fish.

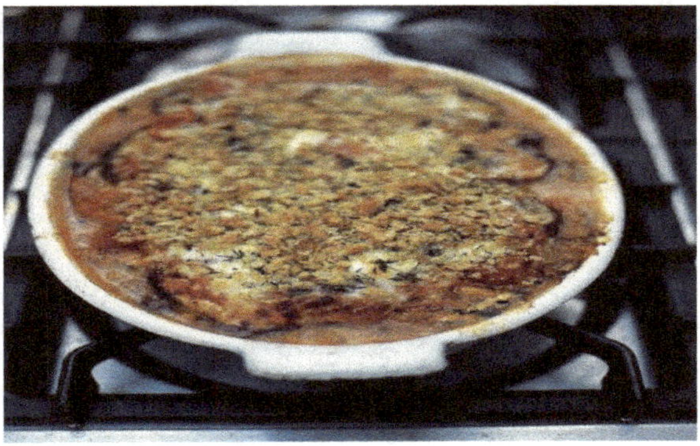

Ingredients

- 1 bunch of fresh basil
- A few sprigs of fresh oregano
- 3 large firm aubergines
- 2 handfuls of dried breadcrumbs
- 150g of buffalo mozzarella
- Olive oil
- ½ a bulb of spring garlic
- 1 heaped teaspoon dried oregano
- 2 x 400g tins of quality plum tomatoes

- Wine vinegar
- 1 onion
- 3 large handfuls of parmesan cheese

Directions

- Preheat a griddle barbecue ready.
- Place a large pan on a medium heat with olive oil.
- Add the onion together with the garlic and dried oregano.
- Let cook for 10 minutes.
- Add the tomato flesh to onion pan, stir well, cover and let simmer 15 minutes over low heat.
- Grill the aubergines on both sides until lightly charred.
- Season the tomato sauce with sea salt, black pepper and a tiny swig of wine vinegar.
- Pick in the basil.
- Spoon a layer of tomato sauce into a baking dish.
- Add a scattering of Parmesan, then single layer of aubergines.
- Repeat these layers until all the ingredients are used.
- Toss chopped oregano with breadcrumbs and some olive oil.
- Sprinkle on top of the Parmesan.
- Tear over the mozzarella.
- Let bake 30 minutes.
- Serve and enjoy.

Bubble and squeak

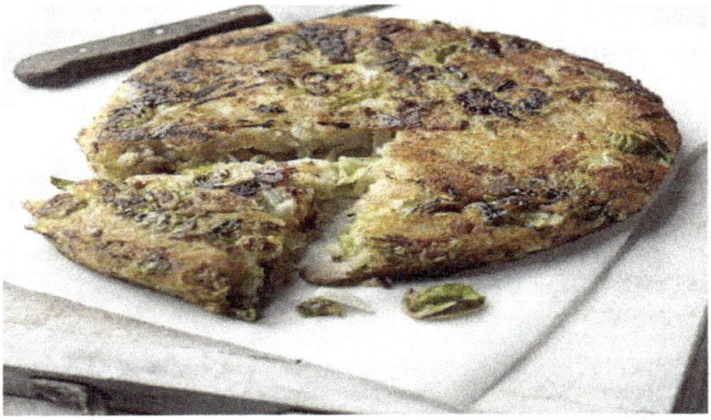

Ingredients

- 600g of leftover cooked vegetables.
- 600g of leftover roast potatoes
- olive oil
- leftover vac-packed chestnuts
- 25g of unsalted butter
- 4 sprigs of fresh woody herbs

Directions

- Place a non-stick frying pan on a medium heat with little olive oil and butter.
- Pick in the fresh herb leaves, let crisp up briefly.
- Add the potatoes, vegetables, and any leftover chestnuts.
- Season with sea salt and black pepper.
- Let cook for 4 minutes or until golden crust forms on the bottom.

- Using a fish slice, fold crispy bits back into the mash.
- Let crisp up again, then repeat the process for 20 minutes.
- Taste and adjust the seasoning accordingly.
- Serve and enjoy with fried eggs and or lemon-dressed watercress.

Speedy quiche tray bake

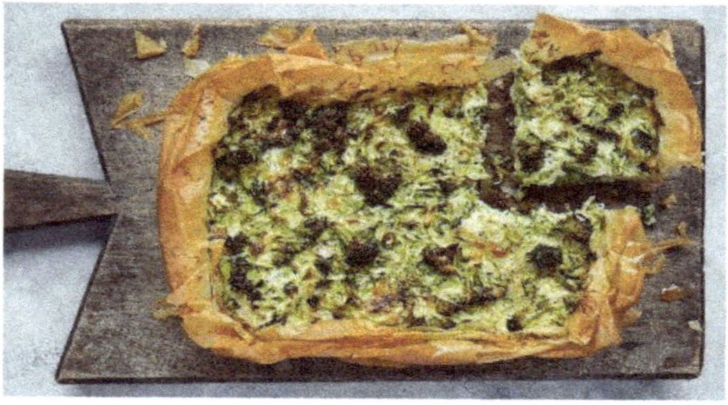

Ingredients

- 6 medium free-range eggs
- 1 x 250g pack of ready-rolled filo pastry
- 55g of mature Cheddar cheese
- 1 large courgette
- 1 bunch of spring onions
- Olive oil
- 300g of broccoli

Directions

- Start by preheating the oven ready to 350°F.
- Then, grease a large roasting tray with bit of olive oil.

- Crack the eggs into a bowl and beat well.
- Layer the filo sheets into the tray, laying one sheet horizontally, and the next vertically, repeating as you layer.
- Bush with bit of egg between each sheet.
- Add a final brush to the last layer and scrunch up any excess pastry.
- Add slice spring onions, cheddar cheese, courgrette, and broccoli to the bowl.
- Season with sea salt and black pepper, mix.
- Pour the mixture into the prepared pastry case, spreading out.
- Sprinkle the remaining cheese over the top.
- Let cook for 35 minutes, until the pastry is golden.
- Serve and enjoy.

Roasted parsnips

This recipe is infused with the acidity of the vinegar that strikes through the entire recipe with bay and honey.

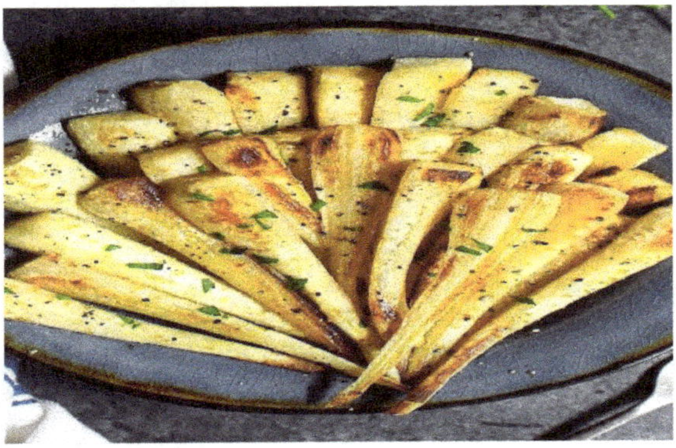

Ingredients

- 4 fresh bay leaves
- 2 tablespoons of runny honey
- 1.5kg of medium parsnips
- 1 tablespoon of white or red wine vinegar
- 50g of unsalted butter

Ingredients

- Firstly, preheat your oven ready to 350°F.
- Blanch whole in a large pan of boiling salted water for 5 minutes.
- Drain off the water and steam dry.
- Tip into a large roasting tray.
- Dot over the butter and a pinch of sea salt and black pepper, toss to coat.
- Organize in a single layer, let roast for at least 1 hour.
- Remove from oven, quickly scatter over the bay leaves.
- Drizzle with the vinegar and honey, toss together.
- Continue to roast for 10 minutes or until golden.
- Serve and enjoy.

Veggie Bolognese sauce

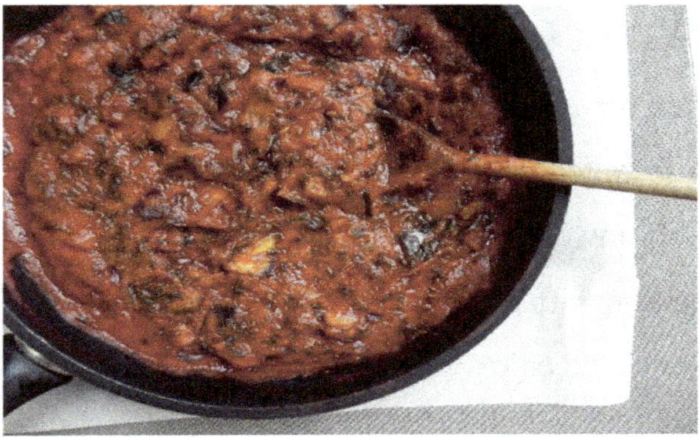

Ingredients

- 250g of alliums
- 1 liter tomato base sauce
- 12g of garlic
- 1 tablespoon of dried mixed herbs
- 1 veggie stock cube
- 750g of Mediterranean veggies
- 25ml of olive oil
- 250g of lentils

Directions

- Place a large pan to hold all the ingredients on a medium heat with the olive oil.
- Add the alliums together with the garlic.
- Let cook for 20 minutes.
- Add the chopped Mediterranean vegetables with the herbs.
- Let cook for 15 minutes or until the vegetables are golden.

- Crush the vegetables.
- Add the lentils with the tomato base sauce, boil.
- Add water and stock cube stir well.
- Boil, lower the heat, let simmer for 40 minutes.
- Season with sea salt and black pepper.
- Serve and enjoy.

Veggie korma

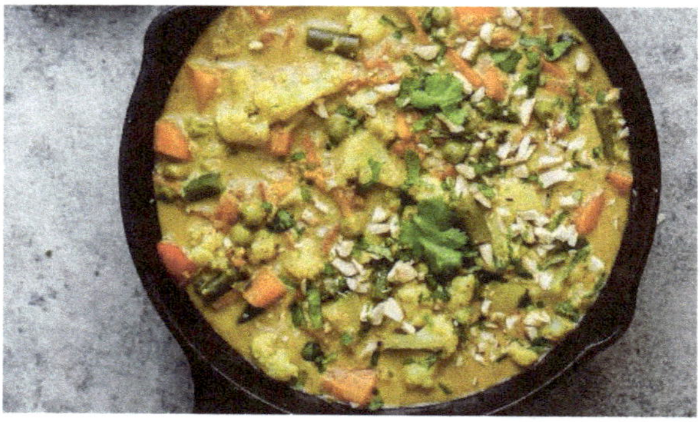

Ingredients

- 2 x 400g tins of chickpeas
- 500g of alliums
- lemon juice
- 175g of plain yoghurt
- 350ml of white base sauce
- 30ml of olive oil
- 2 tablespoons of curry powder
- 2 teaspoons of smoked paprika

- 1kg of mixed vegetables
- 750ml of curry base sauce

Directions

- Place all the ingredients in large a pan over medium heat with the oil.
- Add the alliums together with the curry powder and smoked paprika.
- Cook until the alliums are golden in 20 minutes stirring frequently.
- Add chopped vegetables apart from leafy greens, to the pan, cover let cook briefly.
- Pour in the curry and white sauces with the chickpeas and water.
- Bring to the boil, lower the heat let simmer for 35 minutes.
- Add the reserved leafy vegetables.
- Boil again, let cook until the curry has reduced.
- Stir in the yoghurt until warmed through.
- Season with lemon juice, salt and black pepper.
- Serve and enjoy.

Freezer raid springtime risotto

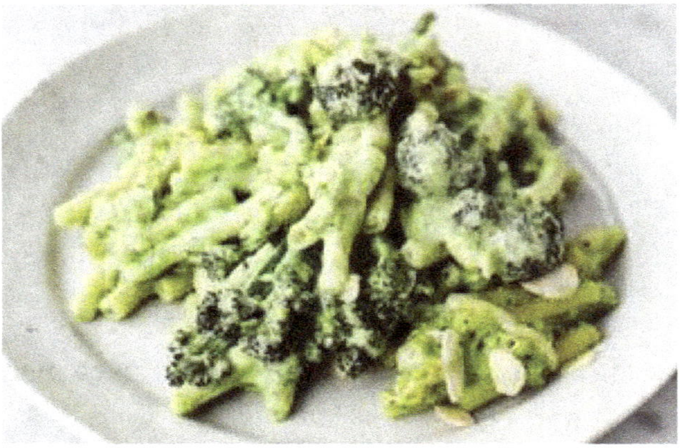

Ingredients

- 300g of mixed frozen green vegetables
- 1 liter of vegetable stock
- Extra virgin olive oil
- 1 onion
- 1 stick of celery
- 60g of freshly grated parmesan cheese
- 1 lemon
- Olive oil
- 2 knobs of unsalted butter
- 300g of risotto rice
- 125ml of white wine

Directions

- Simmer the stock in a pan over a low heat.
- Place 1 tablespoon of olive oil together with knob of butter, onion, and celery into a pan over low heat.

- Season lightly with sea salt and black pepper.
- Cook for 10 minutes, stirring occasionally, until the vegetables are soft.
- Increase the heat to medium.
- Add the rice and stir for 2 minutes, pour in the wine and stir to absorb.
- Add hot stock, stir until fully absorbed, then add more.
- Cook for 18 minutes, adding more stock every minute, stirring regularly.
- Stir in the frozen veggies to cook through 5 minutes to rice cook time.
- Stir in the remaining butter and the Parmesan, season accordingly when heat is off.
- Drizzle with extra virgin olive oil, squeeze in bit of lemon juice per portion.
- Enjoy.

Glazed carrots

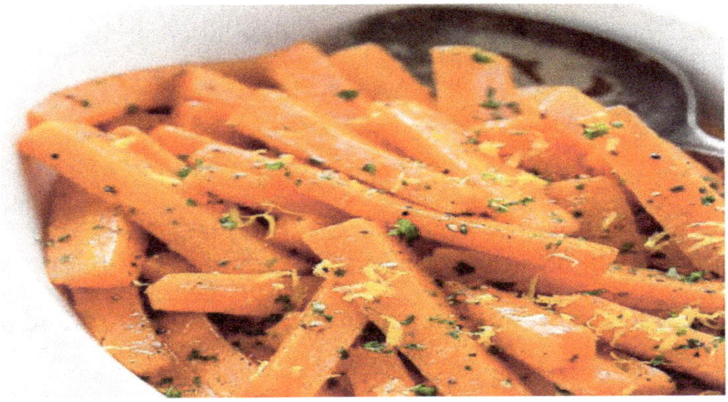

Ingredients

- 50g of unsalted butter
- 2 fresh bay leaves
- 1 tablespoon of dripping
- 2 clementine
- 2 tablespoons of runny honey
- 1kg of small mixed-color carrots
- 6 cloves of garlic
- 8 sprigs of fresh thyme

Directions

- Melt the butter in a large frying pan over a medium heat.
- Add crushed garlic to the pan, turn frequently.
- Sprinkle in the thyme sprigs, clementine juice and honey, bay, and a splash of water.
- Add the carrots, sprinkle with sea salt and black pepper, shake to coat.
- Cover, lower heat to medium-low let cook for 15 minutes.
- Serve and enjoy.

Brussels sprouts

The Brussels sprouts are insanely delicious with apple cubes, Worcestershire and sausages for a great Mediterranean Sea diet.

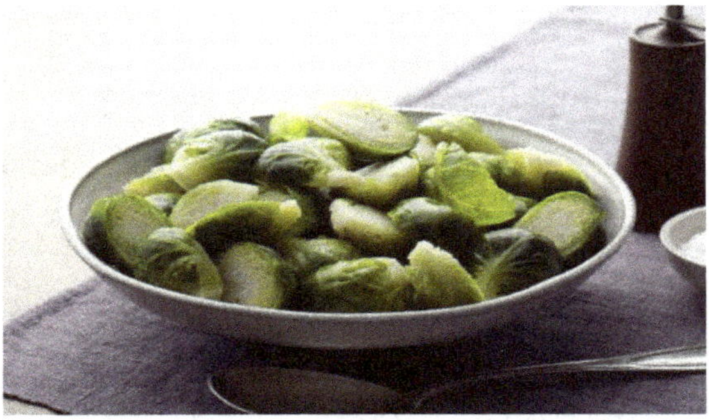

Ingredients

- 1 sweet eating apple
- 1 tablespoon of Worcestershire sauce
- 2 higher-welfare Cumberland sausages
- 1 onion
- 800g of Brussels sprouts
- ½ a bunch of fresh sage
- 20g of unsalted butter

Directions

- Cook the Brussels in a large pan of boiling salted water for 5 minutes.
- Drain any excess water, let steam dry.
- Melt butter in a large frying pan on a medium-low heat.
- Add half the sage leaves and let cook for 3 minutes, transfer into a small bowl.
- Place the pan back on the heat, add the sausage to the pan.
- Cook for 5 minutes, until golden.

- Add the onion with the chopped sage let cook for 5 minutes over medium heat, stirring occasionally.
- Add sliced apples with sprouts, Worcestershire sauce and toss.
- Serve and enjoy with scatter sage leaves on top.

Crispy Moroccan carrots

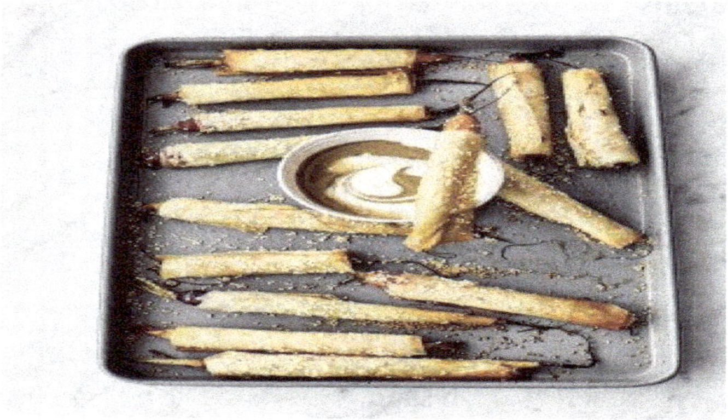

Ingredients

- 6 tablespoons of natural yoghurt
- 12 baby carrots
- Runny honey
- 3 oranges
- 2 teaspoons of rose harissa
- 1 tablespoon of tahini
- 3 fresh bay leaves
- 2 tablespoons of sesame seeds
- 3 sprigs of fresh thyme

- 4 sheets of filo pastry
- Olive oil

Directions

- Preheat the oven ready to 400°F.
- Place and cook the carrots in a pan of fast-boiling salted water for 10 minutes.
- Drain any excess water.
- Grate half the orange zest into the empty pan with all the juice.
- Place on a medium heat.
- Add the bay with thyme and a pinch of sea salt, let cook until syrupy.
- Fold carrots back into the glaze to coat. Let cool.
- Lay out the filo sheets rubbed with oil, then cut lengthways into 3 strips.
- Place a carrot at the bottom of each and roll up.
- Repeat for all the carrots and filo.
- Transfer to a baking tray.
- Brush each lightly with oil, let roast for 20 minutes.
- Drizzle with a little honey and scattering with the sesame seeds for last 5 minutes.
- Stack the carrots on a board, swirl the tahini and harissa through the yoghurt.
- Serve and enjoy.

Rogan josh scotch eggs

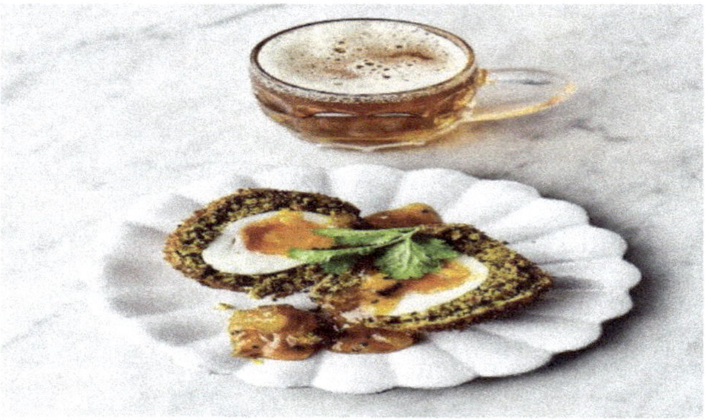

Ingredients

- mango chutney
- 5 large free-range eggs
- 2 liters of vegetable oil
- 2 x 250 g packets of mixed cooked grains
- 50g of plain flour
- 2 heaped teaspoons of Rogan josh curry paste
- 1 bunch of fresh mint
- 1 naan bread

Directions

- Start by soft-boiling 4 eggs in a pan of boiling salted water on a medium heat for 5 minutes.
- Drain, let cool under running water. Peel.
- Place the grains into a food processor with the curry paste, mint leaves, process until tacky in texture.

- Divide into 4 balls.
- Pat one at a time on a greaseproof paper.
- Place the paper flat on your hand, put a peeled egg in the center and mold the mixture up and around the egg to seal it inside.
- Remove the ball from the paper, press in hands to create the perfect covering.
- Place the flour in one bowl, beat the remaining egg in a separate bowl, add the naan to fine crumbs into a third bowl.
- Cover the coated eggs with flour, dip into the beaten egg and roll in the crumbs.
- Place on a medium-high heat.
- Lower the Scotch eggs into the pan let cook for 8 minutes.
- Scoop out and drain on kitchen paper.
- Serve and enjoy.

Moroccan salad with blood oranges, olives, almond and mint

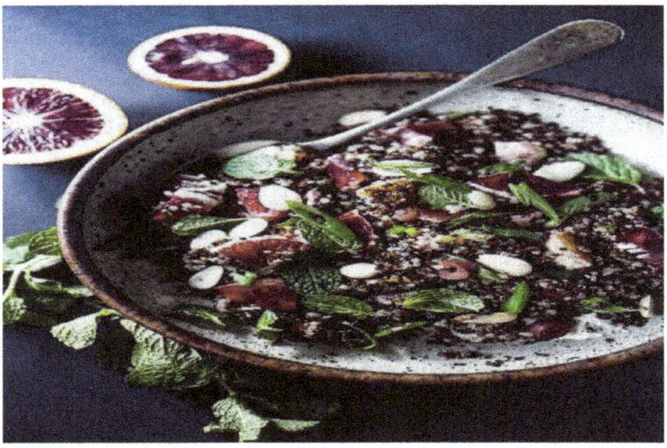

Ingredients

- 1 teaspoon of honey, maple
- 1 ¾ cups of water
- Pinch of salt
- 12 fresh mint leaves, torn
- 2 green onions, sliced diagonally
- 1 tablespoon of red wine vinegar
- 1 cup of rinsed quinoa
- ¼ cup of thinly sliced Kalamata olives
- cracked pepper and salt to taste
- ¼ cup of toasted slivered
- 3 blood oranges- divided
- ¼ cup of olive oil

Directions

- Boil quinoa in salted water in a medium pot on the stove.
- Lower heat once boiling, cover and cook for15 minutes.
- In a medium bowl, add sliced green onions with sliced olives, and 2 oranges.
- Toss the quinoa in the bowl with the oranges.
- Dress with 4 tablespoons of olive oil, zest and juice of the remaining orange, and honey. Stir.
- Taste and adjust accordingly.
- Scatter with toasted slivered almonds and fresh torn mint leaves.

- Serve and enjoy warm or chilled.

Warm grape and radicchio salad

The warm grape and radicchio salad recipe is carefully charred under the grill with incredible fresh balsamic and honey for a sweeter taste.

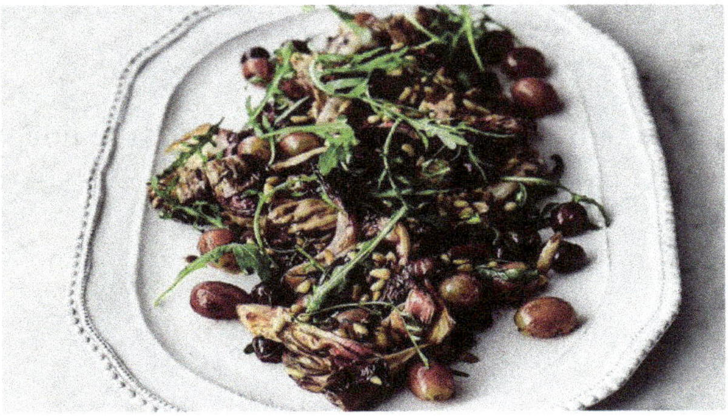

Ingredients

- 30g of rocket
- 200g of seedless red grapes
- 1 radicchio or 2 red chicory
- 1 tablespoon of runny honey
- 2 tablespoons of balsamic vinegar
- Olive oil
- 2 cloves of garlic
- 2 sprigs of fresh rosemary
- 2 heaped tablespoons of pine nuts

Directions

- Place grapes on a griddle pan over a high heat let grill for 5 minutes.
- Transfer in a large salad bowl.
- Working in batches, grill, char the radicchio to soften on both sides.
- Add to the bowl.
- Add garlic, rosemary leaves, pine nuts, and oil in the still-hot griddle pan.
- Add the balsamic vinegar together with the honey. Toss.
- Seasoning with sea salt and black pepper.
- Let settle for 10 minutes, then toss.
- Serve and enjoy.

Nordic nicoise salad

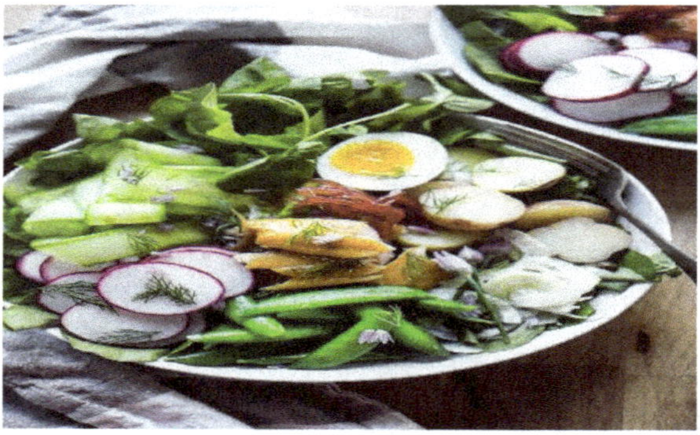

Ingredients

- 2 teaspoons of fresh grated
- 1 tablespoon of chopped fresh dill
- 2 eggs

- 1 cup of snap peas
- 1 cucumber
- Pinch sugar
- 1 tablespoon of finely chopped shallot
- 4 radishes
- 6 ounces of smoked trout
- 1 tablespoon of capers
- 2 tablespoons of fresh dill
- ¼ cup of olive oil
- 2 tablespoons of champagne vinegar
- 8 baby potatoes
- 1 teaspoon of wholegrain mustard
- 1 bunch watercress
- ¼ teaspoon of salt
- ¼ teaspoon of white pepper

Directions

- Boil potatoes, let simmer until tender in 20 minutes.
- Add the snap peas in the same water during the last minute.
- Drain. Rinse under cold water.
- Boil the eggs.
- Stir in olive oil, champagne vinegar, mustard, shallot, dill, salt, sugar, white pepper, and horseradish, tasting and adjust.

- Serve and enjoy with the vegetables salad.

Roasted black bean burgers

The roasted black bean burger features variety of fruits and vegetables typically mango, avocado, tabasco, tomatoes among others, making a perfect Mediterranean Sea diet.

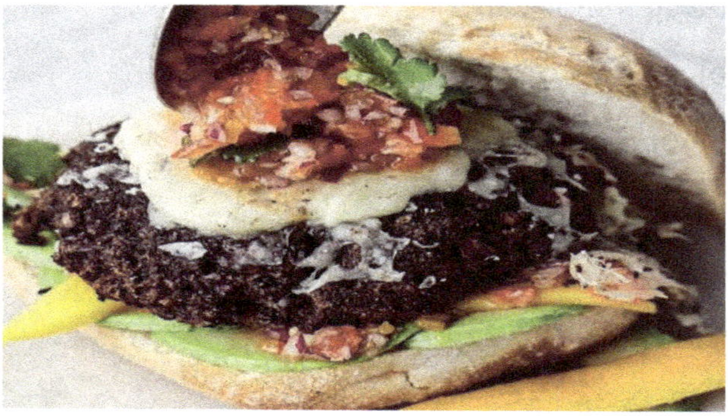

Ingredients

- 1 ripe avocado
- 1½ red onions
- 200g of mixed mushrooms
- Chipotle tabasco sauce
- 4 tablespoons of natural yoghurt
- 100g of rye bread
- Ground coriander
- 1 x 400 g tin of black beans
- 4 sprigs of fresh coriander
- Olive oil

- 40g of mature cheddar cheese
- 1 ripe mango
- 4 soft rolls
- 100g of ripe cherry tomatoes
- 1 lime

Directions

- Preheat the oven ready to 400°F.
- Place 1 onion in a food processor with rye bread mushrooms, and ground coriander process until fine.
- Drain, pulse in the black beans
- Season lightly with sea salt and black pepper.
- Divide into 4 and shape into patties.
- Rub with oil and dust with ground coriander.
- Transfer to oiled baking tray let roast for 25 minutes, until dark and crispy.
- Top with the Cheddar, then warm the rolls.
- Combine the onions and tomatoes in a bowl.
- Squeeze over the lime juice with a bit of Tabasco.
- Season to taste.
- Halve the warm rolls and divide the yoghurt between the bases, and half of the salsa, avocado, mango, and coriander leaves.
- Top with the burgers and the balance of salsa and press down lightly.

- Serve and enjoy.

Brilliant bhaji burger

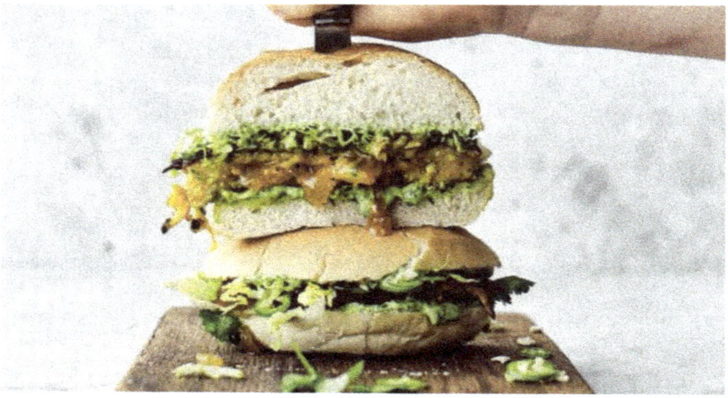

Ingredients

- 2 fresh green chilies
- 75g of paneer cheese
- 200g of butternut squash
- Mango chutney
- 4cm piece of ginger
- 100g of plain flour
- 1 lime
- 2 teaspoons of Rogan josh curry paste
- 2 cloves of garlic
- 2 uncooked poppadum
- Olive oil
- 4 soft burger buns
- 1 red onion

- 1 big bunch of fresh coriander
- 75g of natural yoghurt
- 1 baby gem lettuce

Directions

- Combine onion, garlic, chilies, and coriander stalks in a bowl.
- Add paneer with squash, ginger.
- Sprinkle in the flour and a pinch of sea salt and black pepper.
- Squeeze over the lime juice.
- Add the curry paste and water, mix.
- Drizzle 2 tablespoons of oil into a large non-stick frying pan over a medium heat.
- Divide the mixture into 4 portions and place in the pan.
- Let fry for 16 minutes, turning every few minutes.
- Then pound most of the coriander leaves to a paste in a pestle, muddle in the yoghurt, season.
- Divide the coriander yoghurt between the bases and inside bun-lids, then break up the poppadoms and sprinkle over.
- Place a crispy bhaji burger on top of each bun-base.
- Add a dollop of mango chutney, coriander leaves, and the lettuce.
- Serve and enjoy chilled.

Summer tagliatelle

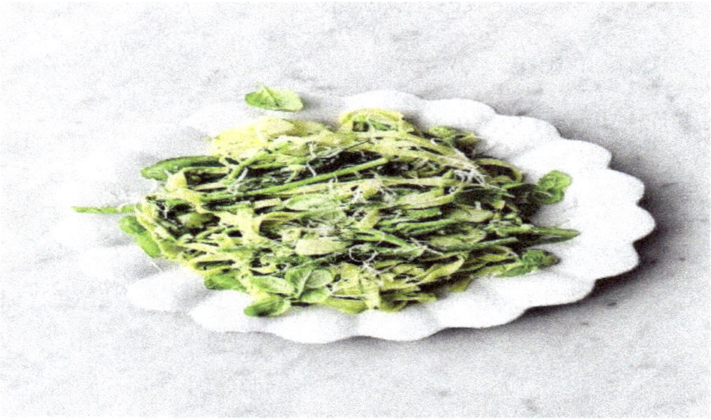

Ingredients

- 1 potato
- ½ a clove of garlic
- 200g of delicate summer vegetables
- 50g of blanched almonds
- 300g of tagliatelle
- Extra virgin olive oil
- 25g of Parmesan cheese
- ¼ of a lemon
- 1 bunch of fresh basil
- 125g of green beans

Directions

- Place most of the basil leaves into a pestle pulse to a paste with a pinch of sea salt.
- Add in the garlic with pounded almonds until fine.

- Muddle in 4 tablespoons of oil with parmesan, squeeze of lemon juice.
- Season accordingly.
- Place sliced potatoes and beans in a pan of boiling salted water with tagliatelle.
- Let cook as per the pasta packet instructions.
- Add delicate summer vegetables to the pan for the last 3 minutes.
- Drain, and keep some cooking water, then toss with the pesto, loosening with a splash of reserved water.
- Drizzle with 1 tablespoon of oil, complete with basil.
- Serve and enjoy with crunchy salad.

Roasted tomato risotto

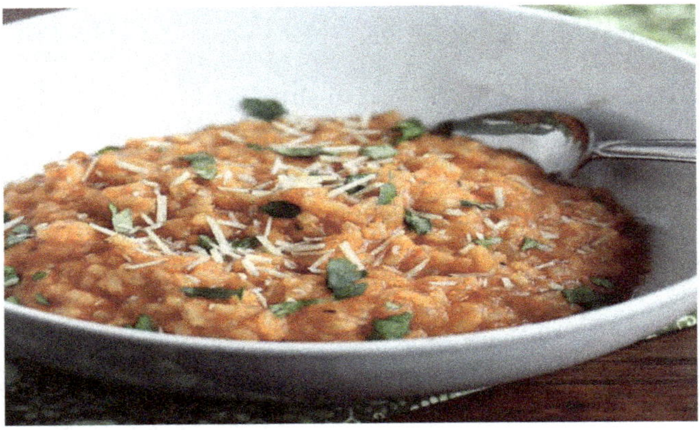

Ingredients

- 450g of Arborio risotto rice
- 80g of Parmesan cheese

- 1 bulb of fennel
- 1 bulb of garlic
- ½ a bunch of fresh thyme
- 150ml of dry white vermouth
- Olive oil
- 1.2 liters of organic vegetable stock
- 1 onion
- 2 knobs of unsalted butter
- 6 large ripe tomatoes

Directions

- Preheat the oven ready to 350°F.
- Remove tomatoes seeds, place in a snug-fitting baking dish with cut sides up with garlic bulb.
- Spread with thyme sprigs.
- Drizzle with 1 tablespoon of oil.
- Season with sea salt, let roast until starting to burst open.
- Bring the stock to a simmer.
- Place onions with olive oil and knob of butter in a large pan on a medium heat. butter.
- Cook until softened, stirring occasionally.
- Stir in the rice, toast for 2 minutes.
- Pour in the vermouth, stir until absorbed.
- Add the stock let it be fully absorbed, then add another, stirring constantly until the rice is cooked in 18 minutes.

- Beat in the remaining knob of butter, Parmesan.
- Season and turn off the heat.
- Let rest for 2 minutes.
- Divide the risotto between warm plates, place a tomato in the center with sweet garlic and the herby fennel.
- Serve and enjoy.

Veggie pad Thai

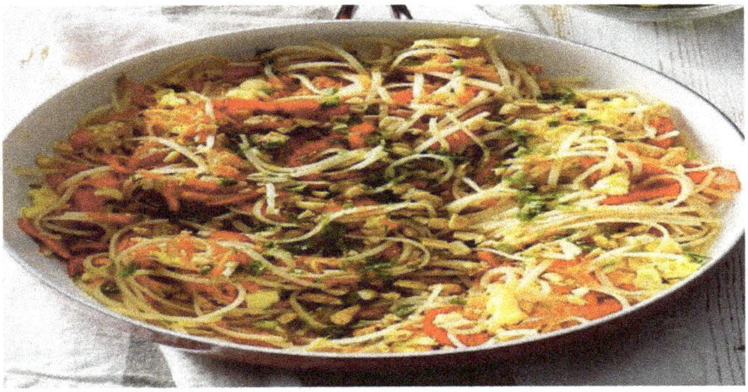

Ingredients

- 320g of crunchy vegetables
- Sesame oil
- Olive oil
- 80g of silken tofu
- Low-salt soy sauce
- 150g of rice noodles
- ½ a mixed bunch of fresh basil, mint and coriander
- 2 teaspoons of tamarind paste
- 2 cloves of garlic

- ½ a cos lettuce
- 2 teaspoons of sweet chili sauce
- 2 limes
- 20g of unsalted peanuts
- 1 shallot
- 80g of beansprouts
- 2 large free-range eggs
- Dried chili flakes

Directions

- Start by cook the noodles according to the packet instructions.
- Drain any excess water, toss with 1 teaspoon of sesame oil.
- Toast the peanuts in a large non-stick frying pan on a medium heat until golden.
- Blend in a pestle until fine, place into a bowl.
- Bash the garlic to a paste with the tofu.
- Add sesame oil with soy, tamarind paste, and chili sauce.
- Muddle in half the lime juice.
- Place slices of shallot in a frying pan over a high heat.
- Dry-fry the crunchy veggies for 4 minutes.
- Add the noodles together with sauce, beansprouts, and splash of water, toss over heat for 1 minute.
- Wipe out the pan, crack in the eggs let cook in a little olive oil, sprinkled with a pinch of chili flakes.

- Place lettuce in the bowls with eggs on top and pick over the herbs.
- Serve and enjoy with lime wedges.

Pea and ricotta stuffed courgettes

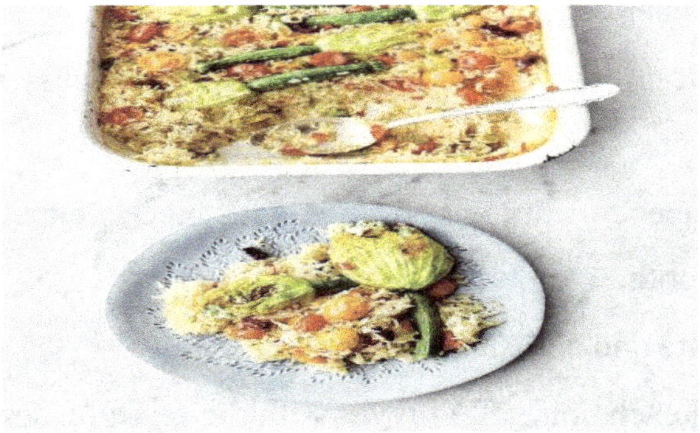

Ingredients

- 2 cloves of garlic
- 4 sprigs of fresh mint
- olive oil
- 100g of ricotta cheese
- 50g of mature Cheddar cheese
- 300g of basmati rice
- 1 lemon
- 8 baby courgettes, with flowers
- 400g of ripe cherry tomatoes
- red wine vinegar
- 150g of fresh or frozen peas

- 4 spring onions
- 8 black olives
- 1 fresh red chili

Directions

- Preheat the oven ready to 400°F.
- Process the mint leaves in a food processor with peas, ricotta, and Cheddar.
- Squeeze in the lemon juice with black pepper, blend until smooth.
- Taste and adjust the seasoning.
- Fill each courgette flower with the mixture, seal the petals.
- Place the tomatoes, onions, and olives roasting tray.
- Drizzle with 2 tablespoons each of oil and vinegar, season with pepper.
- Stir in the rice and boiling water, bring to the boil, stirring occasionally.
- Bake the courgettes inside rice for 20 minutes until golden.
- Serve and enjoy with summery salad

Veggie pasties

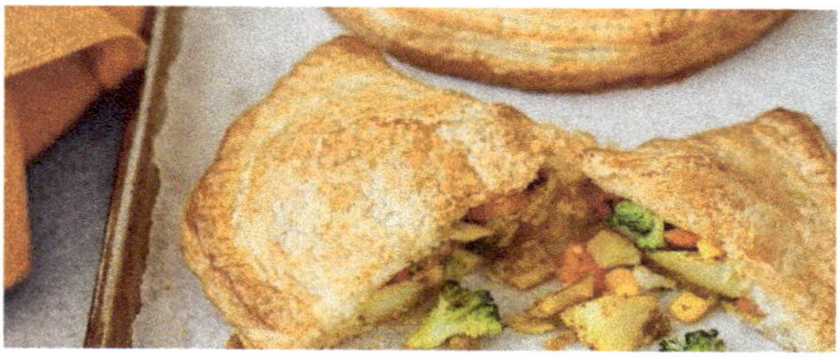

Ingredients

- 1 large free-range egg
- 250g of unsalted butter
- 200g of swede
- 1 pinch of dried rosemary
- 400g of potatoes
- 500g of strong flour
- 1 onion
- 500g of mixed mushrooms

Directions

- Tear the mushrooms into a bowl, scatter over 15g of sea salt, leave for 30 minutes, scrunching occasionally.
- Place flour with a pinch of salt into a bowl.
- Rub in the butter.
- Make a well in the middle, pour in cold water, mix, pat dry.
- Wrap in Clingfilm and refrigerate for 1 hour.
- Squeeze to salty liquid after 30 minutes.
- Mix the veggies with the mushrooms, rosemary and pinches of black pepper.
- Preheat the oven to 350°F.
- Divide the pastry into 8, then roll out into rounds.
- Divide up the filling, then scrunch and pile it to one side of the middle.

- Brush the exposed pastry with beaten egg, fold over and press the edges down, seal with your thumb. Egg wash.
- Place on a lined baking sheet let bake for 40 minutes.
- Serve and enjoy with watercress.

Asparagus quiche and soup

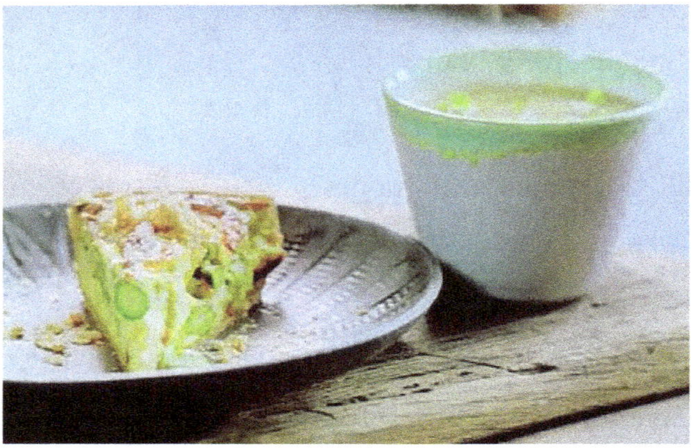

Ingredients

- 1.5 liters of organic vegetable stock
- 125g of whole meal flour
- 2 onions
- 150g of mature Cheddar cheese
- 125g of unsalted butter
- 7 large free-range eggs
- 1kg of asparagus
- 150g of ricotta cheese
- Olive oil

- 125g of plain flour
- 2 large potatoes
- ½ a bunch of fresh thyme

Directions

- Preheat the oven to 350°F.
- Put flours into a bowl with pinch of sea salt, rub in the butter.
- Make a well in the middle, crack in one of the eggs, mix with cold water, pat dry and bring together.
- Place between two large sheets of greaseproof paper, flatten, chill for 30 minutes.
- Roll out the pastry between the sheets, line a loose-bottomed tart tin with the pastry, bake for 20 minutes.
- Place asparagus and oil in a large pan over a medium heat.
- Add the potatoes with onions, thyme leaves cook until lightly golden, stirring regularly.
- Pour in the stock, boil, then simmer for 15 minutes.
- Blend until smooth, sieve.
- Season to taste with salt and black pepper.
- Beat the remaining eggs in a bowl with a pinch of salt and pepper.
- Add the ricotta with Cheddar and remaining thyme leaves.
- Stir the asparagus into the egg mixture and tip into the tart case.
- Let bake for 40 minutes.

- Serve and enjoy.

Summer vegetable blanket pie

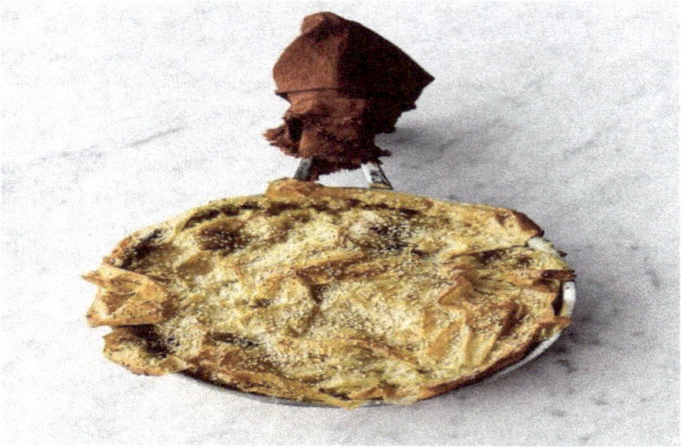

Ingredients

- 320g of ripe cherry tomatoes
- 4 cloves of garlic
- 1 tablespoon of fennel seeds
- Olive oil
- 1 pinch of saffron
- 320g of potatoes
- 320g of butternut squash
- 320g of courgettes
- 1 tablespoon of sesame seeds
- ½ x 700g jar of chickpeas
- 1 large leek
- Extra virgin olive oil

- 8 sheets of filo pastry
- 1 preserved lemon
- 1 tablespoon of red wine vinegar
- 400g of natural yoghurt
- 1 teaspoon of rose harissa
- 50g of dried sour cherries

Directions

- Sieve the yogurt through into a bowl, then leave to drain.
- Season the tomatoes with sea salt and black pepper.
- Drizzle with extra virgin olive oil and the vinegar, then toss, let macerate.
- Preheat the oven to 375°F.
- Place garlic slices in a large frying pan on a medium heat with the fennel seeds and olive oil.
- Fry briefly, stirring regularly.
- Add potatoes, leek, and courgette let cook covered for 15 minutes.
- Add the chickpeas, season with a pinch of salt and pepper.
- Add lemon to the pan with a drizzle of juice from the jar, and the harissa.
- Continue to fry for 15 more minutes, stirring occasionally.
- Cover the sour cherries and saffron with boiling water, add tomatoes, reserving the macerating juices.
- Lay the filo out flat, then brush with tomato juices.

- Scatter over the sesame seeds and bake for 25 minutes
- Serve and enjoy with the pie.

Allotment cottage pie

The delicious taste of the allotment cottage pie will surprise anyone's taste buds. It is fully packed with variety of nutrients and a perfect Mediterranean Sea diet choice.

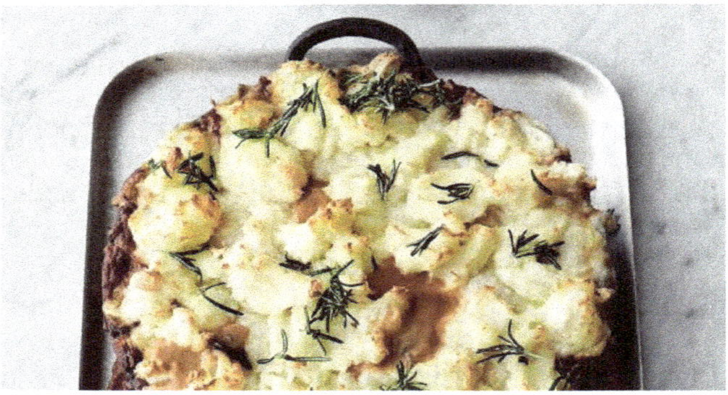

Ingredients

- 1 teaspoon of Marmite
- 2 large leeks
- 3 carrots
- 1 x 400g tin of green lentils
- 1 splash of semi-skimmed milk
- 10g of dried porcini mushrooms
- 500g of swede
- 500g of celeriac
- Olive oil

- 3 sprigs of fresh rosemary
- 1 onion
- 3 tablespoons of tomato purée
- 1 teaspoon cumin seeds
- 2kg of potatoes
- 40g of unsalted butter

Directions

- In a blender, cover the porcini with hot water.
- Drizzle oil into a large casserole pan over a medium heat.
- Fry the rosemary for 1 minute to crisp up.
- Add the cumin seeds together with prepared veggies to flavored oil.
- Season with sea salt and black pepper, cook for 30 minutes, stirring regularly.
- Cook the potatoes in a pan of boiling salted water until tender.
- Drain and mash with butter and milk, then season.
- Preheat the oven to 375°F.
- Add onions, marmite, tomato puree, blend until smooth.
- Pour into the veggie pan and cook for 20 minutes, stirring regularly.
- Place the lentils into the veg pan, boil, season to taste.
- Spoon over the mash, place on a tray.
- Let bake for 30 minutes, or until bubbling at the edges.

- Sprinkle over the crispy rosemary.
- Serve and enjoy with seasonal greens.

Sticky onion tart

The stick onion tart is quite flavorful with garlic and the onion itself. Above and beyond, this recipe is easy to make.

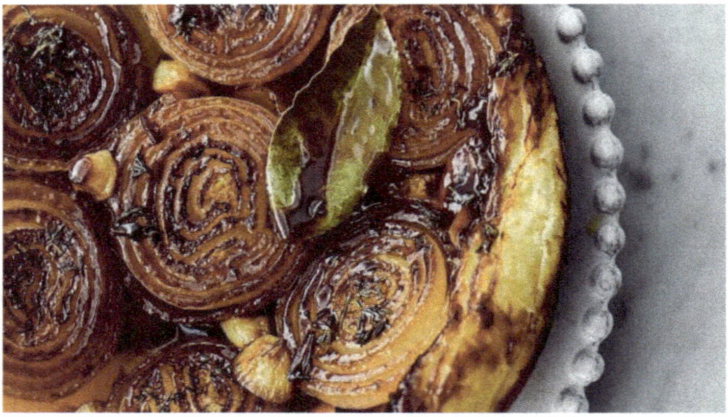

Ingredients

- 4 tablespoons of cider vinegar
- 4 medium onions
- 320g of sheet of all-butter puff pastry
- 50g of unsalted butter
- 8 cloves of garlic
- 4 sprigs of fresh thyme
- 4 fresh bay leaves
- 2 tablespoons of soft dark brown sugar

Directions

- Preheat the oven ready to 425°F.
- Place butter in an ovenproof frying pan on a medium heat.
- Add thyme leaves with the bay, sugar, vinegar, and water.
- Place the onion halves in the pan, cut side down with garlic in between.
- Season with sea salt and black pepper.
- Cover, over low heat and steam for 10 minutes to soften the onions, uncover cook until liquid starts to caramelize.
- Place the pastry over the onions, placed to the edge of the pan.
- Let bake for 35 minutes, until golden brown.
- Serve and enjoy.

Tomato curry

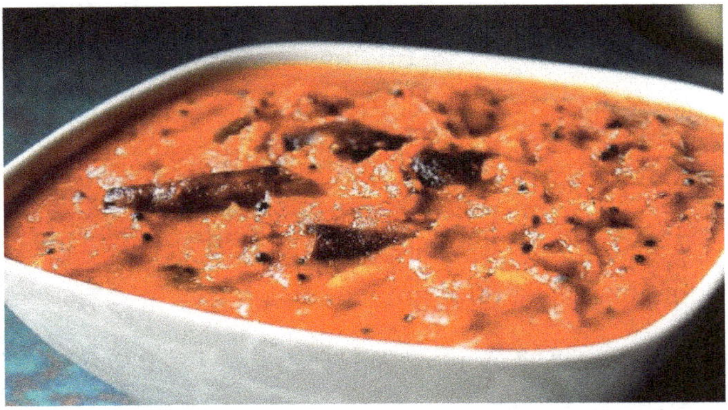

Ingredients

- 2 teaspoons of mango chutney
- 1 onion

- 1.2kg of ripe mixed tomatoes
- 1 pinch of saffron
- 1 teaspoon of mustard seeds
- 1 teaspoon of fenugreek seeds
- 1 x 400g tin of light coconut milk
- 20g of flaked almonds
- 4 cloves of garlic
- 1 teaspoon of cumin seeds
- 4cm piece of ginger
- 2 fresh red chilies
- Olive oil
- 1 handful of fresh curry leaves

Directions

- Prick the tomatoes, plunge into fast-boiling water briefly.
- Peel the skin.
- Cover the saffron with boiling water and leave to infuse.
- Toast the almonds in a large non-stick frying pan over a medium heat until golden.
- Transfer to a small bowl and place the pan back on the heat.
- Drizzle 1 tablespoon of oil into the pan, add curry leaves with all the spices.
- Add onions with garlic, ginger, and chili to the pan, let fry for 3 minutes, stirring constantly.

- Add the tomatoes with the coconut milk and saffron water, let simmer for 20 minutes covered.
- Add mango chutney halfway.
- Season to taste with sea salt and black pepper, scatter over the almonds.
- Serve and enjoy with fluffy rice.

Vegetable chili

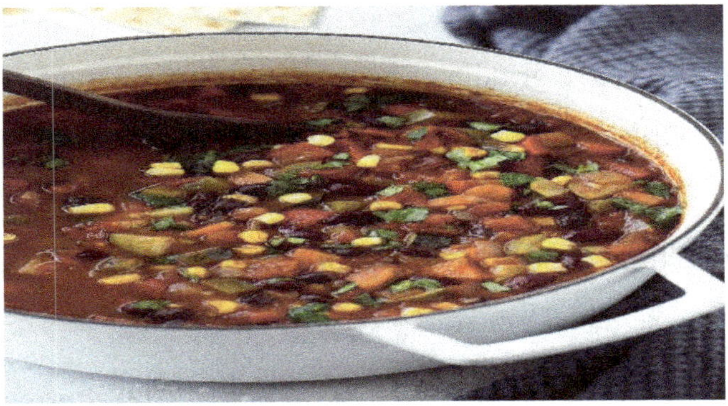

Ingredients

- 2 sweet potatoes
- 1 x 400g tin of cannellini beans
- 3 mixed-color peppers
- 4 large ripe tomatoes
- 1 lemon
- 1 bunch of fresh mint
- 4 tablespoons of natural yoghurt
- Olive oil

- 1 teaspoon of cumin seeds
- 1 teaspoon of smoked paprika
- 2 red onions
- 4 small flour tortillas
- 4 cloves of garlic
- Hot chili sauce
- 250g of black rice

Directions

- Preheat a griddle pan ready to high temperature.
- Drizzle 1 tablespoon of oil into a large casserole pan over a medium-low heat.
- Stir in the cumin with paprika, garlic, lemon zest, and grilled vegetables, stirring regularly.
- Add the beans and water, add chili sauce.
- Season with sea salt and black pepper let simmer for 30 minutes.
- Cook the rice in a pan of boiling salted water according to the packet instructions.
- Pick 2 sprigs of mint leaves and chop with the salsa veggie, toss with the lemon juice.
- Season to taste with salt and pepper.
- Warm the tortillas on the griddle and ripple shakes of chili sauce through the yoghurt.
- Serve and enjoy with black rice.

Chicken and vegetable stir-fry

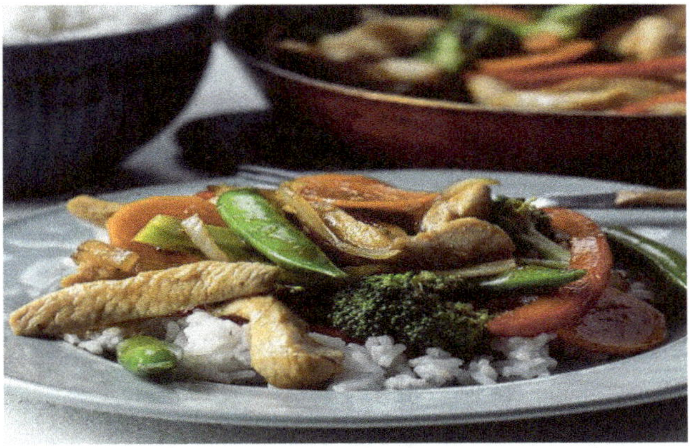

Ingredients

- 2 carrots
- ½ of a red onion
- 1 red pepper
- 80g of purple sprouting broccoli
- 1 tablespoon of reduced-salt soy sauce
- 80g of mixed mushrooms
- 1 free-range chicken breast
- 1 teaspoon of sesame seeds
- 1 tablespoon of sesame oil
- 4cm of piece of ginger
- 1 teaspoon of Chinese five-spice
- 1 teaspoon of vegetable oil
- Sprigs of fresh coriander
- 1 fresh red chili

- 1 clove of garlic
- 130g of baby corn
- 80g of mange tout
- 2 whole wheat noodle nests
- 1 tablespoon of black bean sauce

Directions

- Place the chicken into a bowl with the Chinese five-spice and sesame oil, toss.
- Place a large non-stick frying pan over a medium-high heat with the vegetable oil.
- Add the garlic together with the ginger and chili, toss briefly.
- Add the chicken let stir-fry for 2 minutes until golden.
- Add all the vegetables, let stir-fry for more 4 minutes.
- Cook the noodles as instructed on the package in a large pan of boiling salted water.
- Transfer the noodles to the pan, add soy with black bean sauce, toss to coat.
- Scatter over the sesame seeds and coriander.
- Serve and enjoy.

Roasted vegetable roots

Much as there are various ways one can roast veggies, the Mediterranean style is mega for a delicious and aromatic flavor with garlic taking the lead.

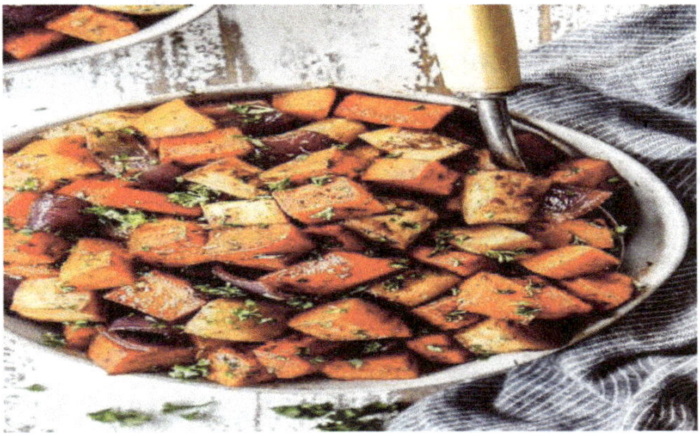

Ingredients

- 12 parsnips
- 3kg of potatoes
- 16 carrots
- ½ a bunch of fresh rosemary
- 1 bulb of garlic

Directions

- Begin by preheat your oven ready to 375°F.
- Cook potatoes with parsnips and carrots in a large pan of boiling salted water for 8 minutes.
- Drain any excess water in a colander let steam dry.
- Remove the carrots and parsnips put to one side, shakes the colander.
- Add 4 tablespoons of olive oil to two large roasting trays.
- Season each with sea salt and black pepper.

- Squash the garlic bulb, divide between the trays with the rosemary sprigs.
- Place in the veggies, red wine vinegar, toss to coat.
- Let roast for 40 minutes.
- Remove and squash with a fish slice to burst the skins.
- Place back in the oven for 20 minutes.
- Serve and enjoy.

Beetroot curry

What a blessing to add onto your body blood. Beet root is a gift to replenish blood in the body; as such, this recipe cannot be underestimated among Mediterranean Sea diets with earthly flavors.

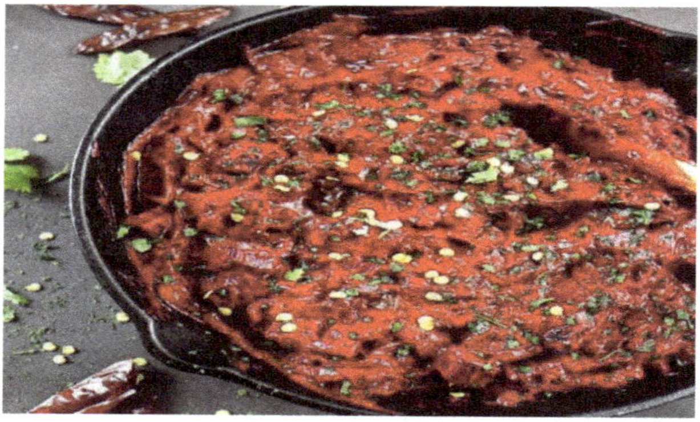

Ingredients

- 1 teaspoon of hot curry powder
- 3 cloves of garlic
- 2 tablespoons of desiccated coconut
- 3 cloves of garlic

- 5cm of piece of ginger
- vegetable oil
- 2 teaspoons of black mustard seeds
- 1 kg mixed beets
- 250g of ripe cherry tomatoes
- 7g of dried curry leaves
- ½ a bunch of fresh coriander
- 320g of wild rice
- 6 spring onions
- 14g of dried curry leaves
- 5cm of piece of ginger
- 1 x 400ml tin of light coconut milk
- 1 lemon
- 1 lime
- 2 fresh long red chilies

Directions

- Place a large pan over a medium heat.
- Add the curry leaves with the curry powder, mustard seeds, and coconut, let toast for 2 minute. Transfer to a food processor and blend well.
- Add spring onions to the food processor with garlic, ginger, and vegetable oil.
- Pulse to forms a paste.
- Place the pan back on the hob over a medium heat.

- Add the paste cook briefly, add beetroot.
- Lower heat and cook until sticky and gnarly, stirring often.
- Add the cherry tomatoes and cook for 5 minutes, then break them with the back of a spoon.
- Cook the rice as instructed on the packet.
- Stir in the coconut milk with a squeeze of lemon juice.
- Raise the heat let cook for 5 minutes.
- Season to taste.
- Place a frying pan over a medium heat with oil.
- Add all the temper ingredients let heat for 2 minutes.
- Turn off the heat, transfer into a bowl lined with kitchen paper.
- Serve the curry with the rice and temper and or coriander leaves scattered on top.
- Serve and enjoy.

Brick lane burger

Everyone likes to enjoy a delicious burger, isn't it? If yes, then this Mediterranean Sea diet recipe is a must try for you. It has great flavors derived from onions, garlic and ginger.

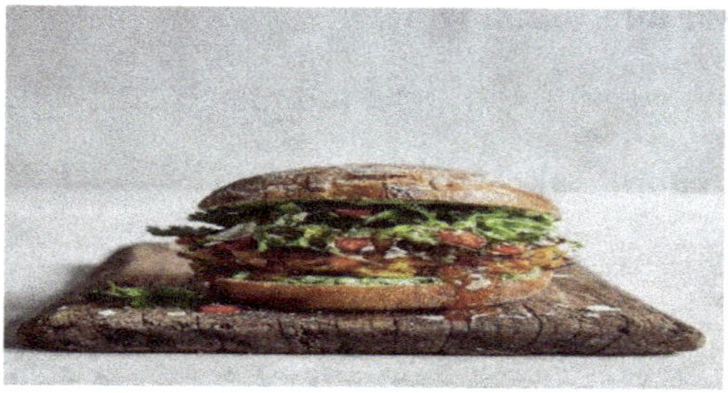

Ingredients

- 200g of butternut squash
- 2 cloves of garlic
- 2 fresh green chilies
- 100g of paneer cheese
- Mango chutney
- 1 big bunch of fresh coriander
- 150g of gram flour
- 6 burger buns
- 2 teaspoons of ground turmeric
- 3 poppadoms
- 2 baby gem lettuce
- 1 carrot
- 2 teaspoons of ground cumin
- 2 red onions
- 2 limes
- Olive oil
- 100ml of natural yoghurt
- 5cm of piece of ginger
- 1 fresh red chili

Directions

- Preheat the oven to 350°F.

- Place onions, carrots, paneer, garlic, ginger, and coriander into a large mixing bowl.
- Place flour together with the turmeric and cumin.
- Season with sea salt and black pepper, squeeze in the juice of 1 lime with water, mix with your hands.
- Divide into 6, then shape and squash into patties.
- Drizzle with bit of oil into a large non-stick frying pan over a medium heat.
- Let fry the patties for 3 minutes on each side or until golden.
- Remove to a baking tray for 10 minutes or until cooked.
- Pestle the remaining coriander leaves, setting aside a handful.
- Add a pinch of salt, then bash to a paste. Squeeze in the juice of lime, stir in the yoghurt.
- Spoon a little coriander yoghurt over the base and inside lid of each burger bun.
- Crumble the poppadoms, sprinkle over the yoghurt, then sit a patty on top of each base and spread with 1 tablespoon of mango chutney.
- Top with a handful of lettuce and the reserved coriander leaves.
- Sprinkle with red chili
- Serve and enjoy.

Summer vegetable lasagna

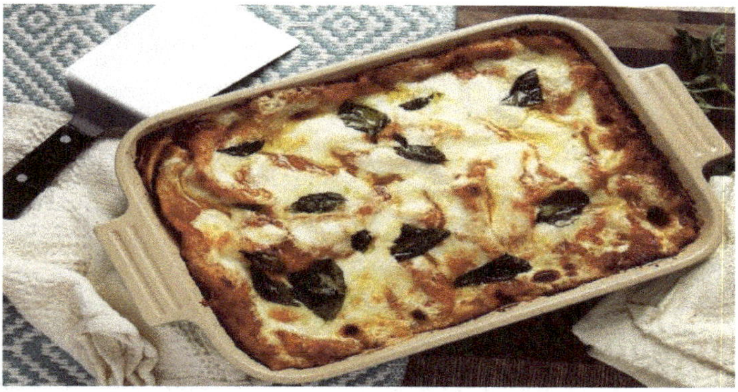

Ingredients

- Olive oil
- ½ x 30g tin of anchovies in oil
- 6 cloves of garlic
- 500g of fresh lasagne sheets
- 700g of asparagus
- 1 lemon
- Sprigs of fresh thyme
- 500g of frozen peas
- 300g of frozen broad beans
- Parmesan cheese
- 1 bunch of spring onions
- 1 big bunch of fresh mint
- 300ml of single cream
- 300m of organic vegetable stock
- 2 x 250g tubs of cottage cheese

Directions

- Preheat the grill to full temperature.
- Pour oil from the anchovy tin into a large frying pan over a high heat
- Add the spring onions and anchovies.
- Add crushed garlic, toss well.
- Add asparagus stems to the pan, keep tips for later.
- Season with sea salt and black pepper.
- Add a splash of boiling water, let cook for a few minutes, stirring occasionally.
- Add the peas together with the broad beans, mint, lemon zest, and the cream to the pan.
- Squash, then season with salt and pepper.
- Pour in the stock and bring to the boil.
- Stir in 1 tub of cottage cheese.
- Place a roasting tray over a medium heat.
- Cover the bottom of the tray with the vegetable mixture, then top with a layer of lasagne sheets, and Parmesan grating.
- Repeat the layers with the rest of the vegetable mixture and pasta, use lasagne sheets to finish.
- Mix the remaining tub of cottage cheese with splash of water.
- Toss the reserved asparagus with a drizzle of oil.
- Strip over the thyme leaves.

- Turn the heat under the tray up to high and cook until the lasagne starts to bubble, place under the grill on the middle shelf for 8 minutes.
- Serve and enjoy.

Gnarly cauliflower curry

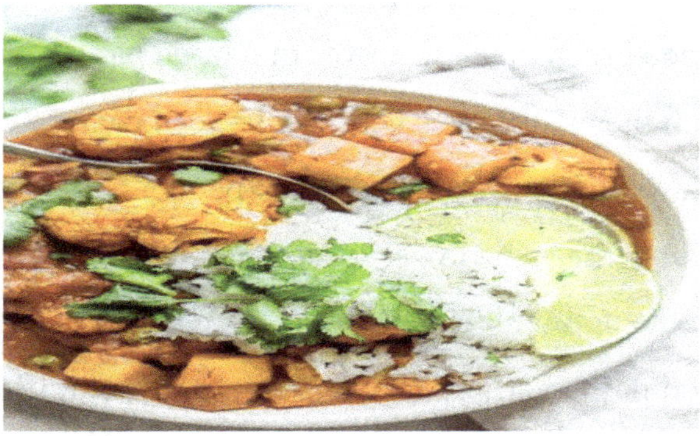

Ingredients

- ½ x 400g tin of light coconut milk
- 1 medium cauliflower
- 2 heaped tablespoons of rogan josh curry paste
- Extra virgin olive oil
- 2 heaped tablespoons of natural yoghurt
- 1 red onion
- 1 pinch of dried red chili flakes
- 2 cloves of garlic
- 150g of basmati rice
- 2 lemons

- 4 uncooked poppadoms
- ½ a bunch of fresh coriander
- Pickled chilies

Directions

- Preheat the grill to high.
- Place prepared cauliflower in a large pan.
- Rub the cauliflower with Rogan josh paste.
- Season with sea salt and black pepper.
- Add in the cauliflower leaves then place over a medium heat on the hob with water.
- Add in the garlic, onions, on top of the cauliflower.
- Bring to the boil, let bubble for 10 minutes.
- Transfer the pan to the grill, 5cm away, for 15 minutes or until gnarly, charred and cooked through.
- Cook the rice in a pan of boiling salted water per the packet instruction with half a lemon, drain excess water.
- Pick the coriander leaves from 1 sprig and scatter over with a few pickled chilies and liquor. Mix.
- Drizzle with 1 tablespoon of oil.
- Remove the cauliflower, place over a medium heat.
- Pour in the coconut milk let boil, stirring gently.
- One-by-one, puff up your dry poppadoms in the microwave briefly.

- Add coriander stalks to a pestle with a pinch of salt and chili flakes blend to a paste.
- Muddle in the yoghurt.
- Sprinkle the coriander leaves over the curry, add lemon into rice.
- Serve and enjoy with poppadoms, and lemon pickle.

Pot roasted cauliflower

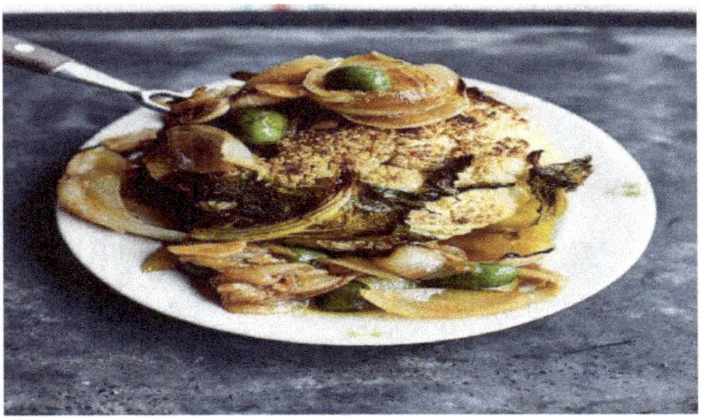

Ingredients

- 1 small pinch of saffron
- Olive oil
- 1 large head of cauliflower
- 6 cloves of garlic
- 3 onions
- 6 large green olives
- 6 anchovy fillets in oil
- 500ml of white wine

Directions

- Preheat the oven to 350°F.
- Combine onions, olive oil, and anchovies in an ovenproof pan on a medium-high heat.
- Add olive with the garlic let cook for 2 minutes, pour in the wine with saffron.
- Sit the cauliflower in the pan, stalk side down.
- Drizzle with 1 tablespoon of oil.
- Spoon bit of onions and liquid over the cauliflower, boil.
- Transfer the pan to the oven for 1 hour.
- Carefully lift the cauliflower on to a platter and spoon over the soft onions, olives and fragrant juices from the pan.
- Serve and enjoy with sliced onions and olives.

Peas, beans, chili and mint

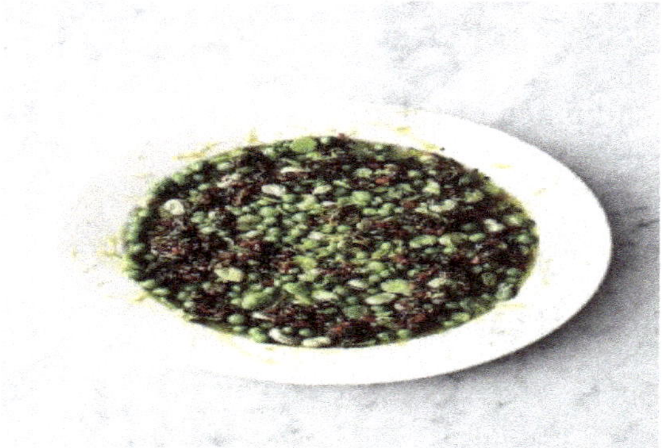

Ingredients

- 1 lemon

- 1 fresh red chili
- 200g of fresh podded
- ½ a bunch of fresh mint
- 200g of fresh podded

Directions

- Put the mint stalks in a pan of boiling salted water, with the beans and peas to cook for 4 minutes.
- Combine leafy mint, lemon zest, extra virgin oil, and chili in a bowl, mix.
- Season with sea salt and black pepper.
- Drain the beans and peas, reserving some cooking water for later.
- Pinch the skins off any larger beans, pour the beans and peas on to a platter, toss with a few splashes of reserved cooking water, then spoon over the dressing.
- Drizzle with extra virgin olive oil and toss together.
- Serve and enjoy.

Dressed beets

This recipe embraces the healthy benefits of beets, citrus, vinegar and walnuts for a perfect Mediterranean Sea diet.

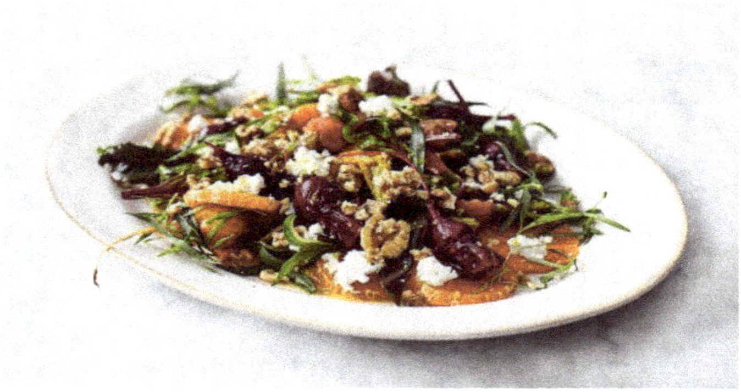

Ingredients

- 100g of crumbly goat's cheese
- 4 clementine
- 600g of raw mixed-color baby beets
- 40g of shelled unsalted walnut halves
- Extra virgin olive oil
- Red wine vinegar
- ½ a bunch of fresh tarragon

Directions

- Cook the beets covered, in a pan of boiling salted water for 20 minutes.
- Squeeze the juice of 1 clementine into a large bowl with extra virgin olive oil and red wine vinegar.
- Slice and arrange remaining clementine on a plates.
- Drain the beets rub off the skins when cooled under running water.

- Season with sea salt and black pepper, add the tarragon and toss with the reserved beet leaves.
- Divide between your plates, crumble over the goat's cheese and walnuts.
- Serve an enjoy drizzled with extra virgin olive oil.

Roasted roots halloumi tray bake with courgette tangles

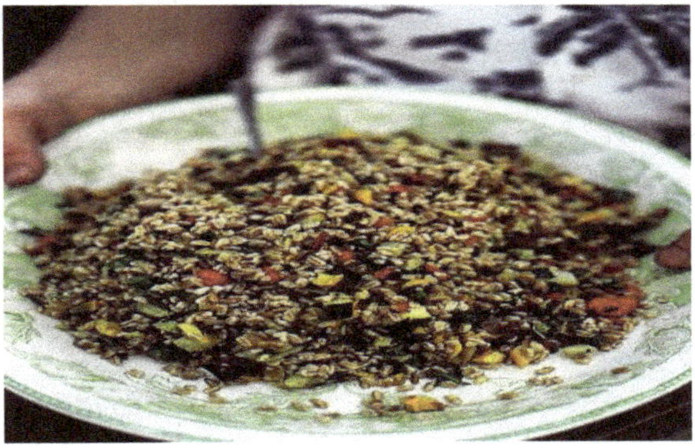

Ingredients

- 4 tablespoons of quality green pesto
- 1 small broccoli
- Olive oil
- 800g of mixed root veggies
- 250g of halloumi cheese
- 2 red peppers
- 1 large eating apple
- 1 courgette
- 100g of lamb's lettuce

Directions

- Preheat the oven to 400°F.
- Spread the veg out on a large roasting tray.
- Drizzle with olive oil.
- Then, season with sea salt and black pepper, toss to coat.
- Let roast until the vegetables are tender and colored.
- Cut and scatter over the veggies.
- Switch the oven to grill, raise the heat and grill for 10 minutes.
- Spiralize the courgette.
- Combine sliced apple with the roasted veggies, then stir through the courgette and spinach.
- Mix the pesto with 2 tablespoons of oil and drizzle over.
- Serve and enjoy.

Parsnip beetroot gratin

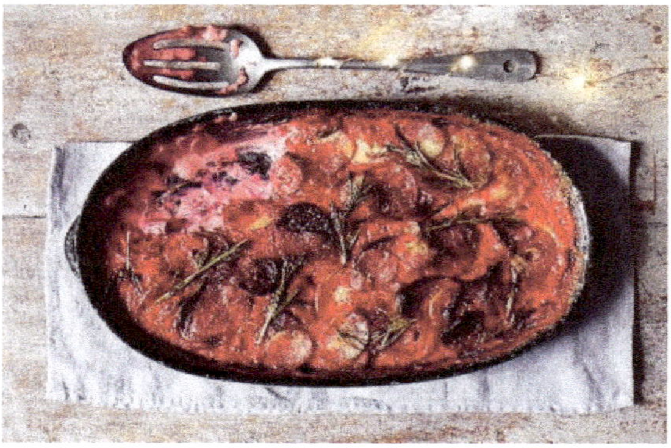

Ingredients

- 2 oranges
- 500g of beetroots
- 300ml of double cream
- Unsalted butter
- ½ a bunch of fresh rosemary
- 200ml of crème fraiche
- 500g of parsnips
- 4 cloves of garlic

Directions

- Preheat the oven to 400°F.
- Oil a 1.5-liter baking dish ready.
- Layer up sliced parsnips and beets in the baking dish.
- Put the cream together with the crème fraiche, whole unpeeled garlic, and rosemary sprigs in a saucepan, let simmer.
- Remove the heat, add orange zest.
- Season with sea salt and a big pinch of black pepper.
- Pour the cream over the vegetables, pressing them to submerge in the liquid and arrange the rosemary sprigs on top.
- Cover tightly with tin foil
- Let bake for 45 minutes, until the vegetable is almost tender.
- Remove the foil and continue to bake for 25 minutes.
- Cool for 5 minutes.

- Serve and enjoy.

Roasted radish and runner bean tray bake

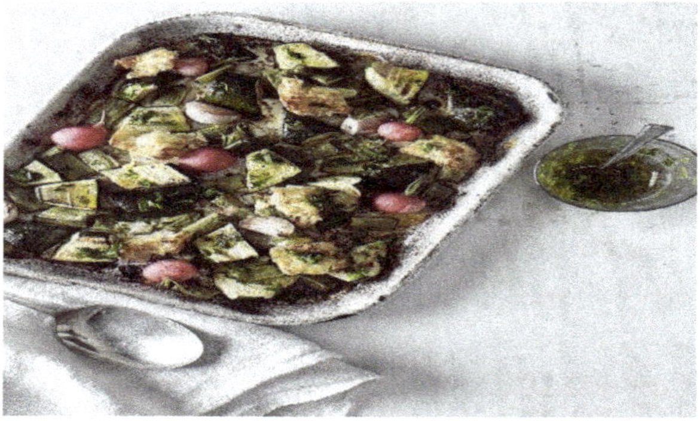

Ingredients

- 25g of Cheddar cheese
- 1 tablespoon of red wine vinegar
- 150g of runner beans
- 70g of ciabatta
- Sprigs of fresh dill, flat-leaf parsley, chives
- 6 radishes, with tops
- 3 cloves of garlic
- 1 teaspoon of runny honey
- 100ml of white wine
- 2 courgettes
- Olive oil
- Extra virgin olive oil

Directions

- Preheat the oven to 375°F.
- Pour in the wine or stock.
- Season with sea salt and black pepper, drizzle over 2 tablespoons of olive oil.
- Coarsely blend the cheddar and sprinkle over the bread pieces.
- Let roast in the oven for 40 minutes or until cooked through.
- Combine 2 tablespoons of extra virgin olive oil with the honey and vinegar.
- Stir through the chopped herbs, season and keep aside.
- Remove the tray from the oven and drizzle with the dressing.
- Serve and enjoy on a bed of spinach.

Apricot, root veggie cake with honey yogurt icing

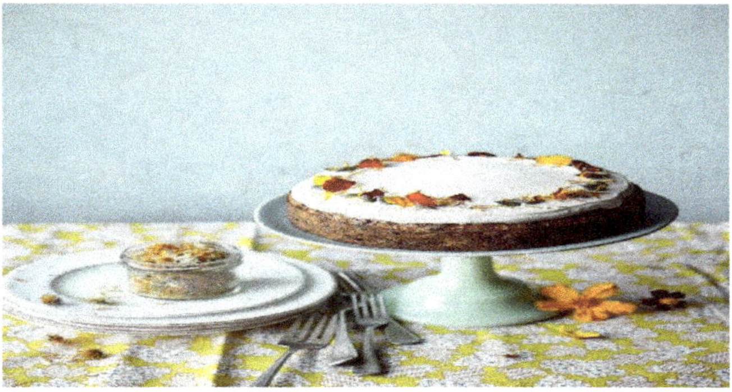

Ingredients

- 150g of Greek-style natural yoghurt
- 40g of pumpkin seeds
- 1 beetroot

- 2 parsnips
- 1 orange
- 1 lemon
- 120g of quality maple syrup
- 2 large free-range eggs
- 25g of clear runny honey
- 70 ml cold-pressed rapeseed oil
- 150g of wholegrain spelt flour
- 1 pinch of mixed spice
- 2 medium carrots
- 1 teaspoon baking powder
- 60g of dried apricots
- 150g of cream cheese
- ½ teaspoon of quality vanilla extract

Directions

- Preheat the oven to 350°F.
- Oil the base and sides of a loose-bottomed cake tin with a little rapeseed oil.
- Line the base with baking paper.
- Grate and combine the carrots, beetroot and parsnip into a large bowl.
- Add grated zest of the orange and 2/3 to the veggie with maple syrup, eggs, and rapeseed oil.
- Fold in the flour, spice, baking powder and a pinch of salt.

- Add diced apricot with seeds to the bowl, Mix to combine.
- Pour the mixture into the prepared tin let bake for 40 minutes, rotating the tin after 20 minutes.
- Let cool in the tin.
- Whisk together all the ingredients except the lemon, until smooth.
- Squeeze in a tiny bit of lemon juice and whisk again.
- Chill in the fridge until needed.
- Transfer to a plate finish with the icing.
- Slice and enjoy.

Roasted sprouts

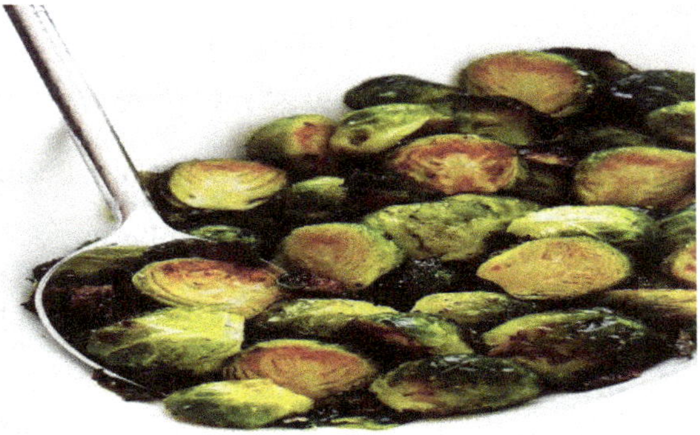

Ingredients

- 1 small clove of garlic
- 500g of Brussels sprouts
- 1 lemon
- 25g of hazelnuts

- 2 teaspoons of coriander seeds
- 1 heaped teaspoon of tahini
- 2 small red onions
- ½ a bunch of fresh coriander
- 1 bulb of fennel
- Olive oil
- 1 pinch of sumac
- 1 teaspoon of sesame seeds
- 1 teaspoon of cumin seeds
- 200g of Greek yoghurt

Directions

- Preheat the oven to 400°F.
- Boil water salted in a large pan over a medium-high heat.
- Add sprouts to the pan let boil for 3 minutes.
- Drain excess water in a colander let dry.
- Toast the cumin together with the coriander seeds in a small frying pan over a medium heat until fragrant.
- Grind the toasted seeds with a pinch of sea salt using a mortar.
- Add the spice mix into a large roasting tray and toss with sprouts.
- Add onions into the tray with bit of oil.
- Spread everything in an even layer then, cook for 20 minutes.

- Return the frying pan to the heat and toast the sesame seeds together with the hazelnuts for 3 minutes.
- Grind up with the remaining spices, using a mortar.
- Combine the yoghurt with the tahini.
- Stir the crushed garlic through with lemon zest juice.
- Taste the yoghurt and season accordingly.
- Spread over the base of a large serving platter sprinkled with sumac.
- Spoon the sprout mix on top of the yoghurt mixture.
- Sprinkle the ground nuts and seeds over the top.
- Serve and enjoy with herb leaves scattered on the plate.

Whole roasted miso aubergine

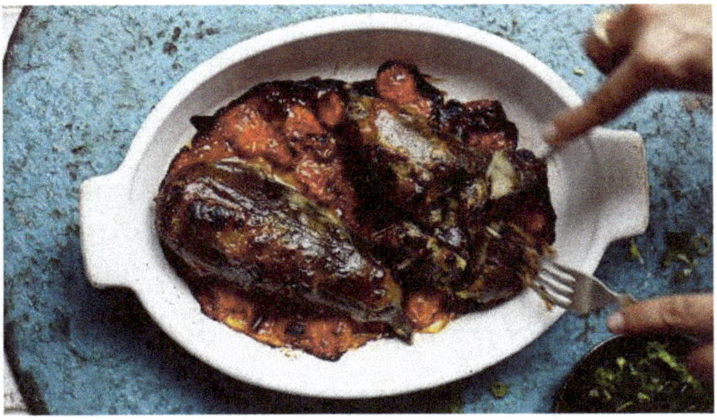

Ingredients

- 1 tablespoon of tamarind paste
- 4 cloves of garlic
- 3 tablespoons of white sweet miso

- 2 small green chilies
- groundnut oil
- 200g of vine cherry tomatoes
- 3cm piece of ginger
- 4 spring onion
- ½ a bunch of coriander
- 1 lime
- 2 aubergines
- ½ tablespoon of honey

Directions

- Preheat your oven ready to 350°F.
- Grate the ginger into a large mortar and pestle, combine together with the garlic, chilies, and a pinch of salt, mix to form a thick paste.
- Spoon the mixture over the aubergines and massage it into the incisions on the meat.
- Place the aubergines in a large roasting tray.
- Dot the cherry tomatoes place into the oven for 40 minutes, turning occasionally.
- While the aubergines are cooking, trim and finely slice the spring onions and roughly chop the coriander, stalks and all. Add the onions together with the coriander stalks, squeeze over the lime juice to coat and mix well.
- Combine the tamarind with honey, miso, and water.

- Remove the roasting tray from the oven after 40 minutes.
- Raise the heat to high then drizzle the miso glaze over the aubergines.
- Return back into the oven for more 15 minutes.
- Remove the stalks from the aubergines and throw away.
- Chop the flesh in the tray into coarse chunks.
- Stir in the dressed spring onions.
- Serve and enjoy.

Roasted brassicas with puy lentil and halloumi

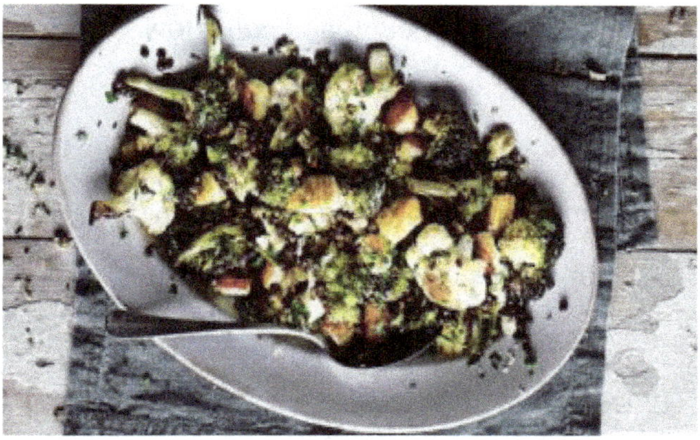

Ingredients

- 1 large bunch of mixed soft herbs
- Olive oil
- 1 heaped teaspoon of baharat
- 2 tablespoons of runny honey
- 4 cloves of garlic
- 250g of puy lentils

- 250g of halloumi cheese
- 1 liter of organic vegetable stock
- 800g of broccoli and cauliflower
- 1 fresh bay leaf
- 2 lemons
- Extra virgin olive oil
- 100g of walnuts

Direction

- Preheat the oven to 425°F.
- Spread out the broccoli and cauliflower in a single layer in a roasting tray.
- Drizzle with olive oil, then sprinkle with Baharat.
- Season with sea salt and black pepper.
- Toss in cloves of garlic, spread out in the tray.
- Roast for 25 minutes.
- Place lentils in a medium-sized pan.
- Pour over the hot stock, add the bay leaf.
- Boil over a medium heat, lower heat let simmer and cook for 30 minutes. Drain and set aside.
- Mash the garlic until creamy, add lemon juice let season and extra virgin olive oil. Season.
- Toast the walnuts with the herb leaves. Keep aside.
- Toss the hot lentils through the garlic dressing, with roasted veggies, herbs and nuts.

- Pour olive oil into a medium-sized, non-stick frying pan over a medium heat, fry the halloumi till golden.
- Drizzle with honey and fry for briefly.
- Serve and enjoy.

Lentil tabbouleh

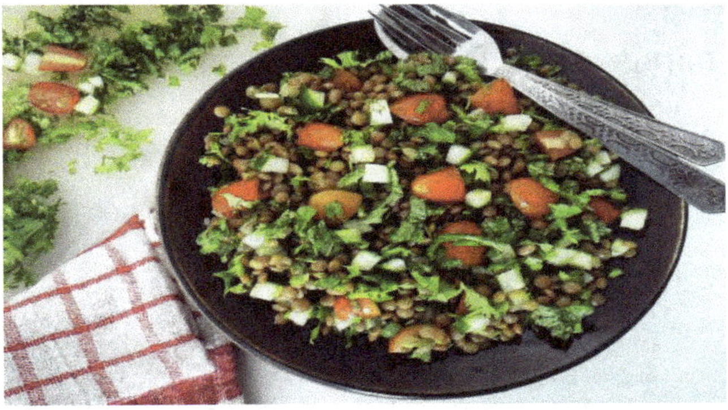

Ingredients

- 1 lemon
- Extra virgin olive oil
- 1 bunch of spring onions
- 1 large bunch of fresh mint
- 200g of ripe cherry tomatoes
- 200g of lentils
- 1 large bunch of fresh flat-leaf parsley

Directions

- Cook the lentils in plenty of salted water until tender.

- Drain any excess water and set aside to cool.
- Mix the cooled lentils together with the tomatoes, spring onions, herbs, and 4 tablespoons of oil.
- Add the lemon juice.
- Season with sea salt and black pepper.
- Serve and enjoy.

Fresh mango salsa

The Mediterranean mango recipe is quite easy to make is few minutes. The colorful spicy salad is remarkable delicious especially when served with chips on tacos.

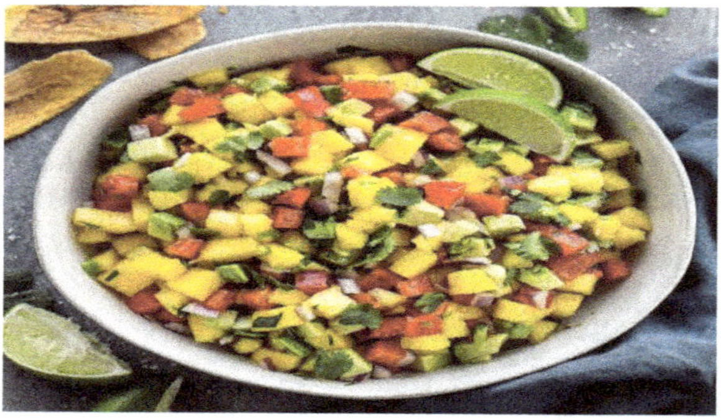

Ingredients

- 1 jalapeño, seeded and minced
- ¼ teaspoon salt, to taste
- 1 medium red bell pepper
- ½ cup of chopped red onion
- 3 ripe mangos

- 1 large lime, juiced
- ¼ cup of packed fresh cilantro leaves

Directions

- In a serving bowl, combine the prepared mango with bell pepper, onion, cilantro, and jalapeño.
- Drizzle with the juice of 1 lime.
- Stir the ingredients together.
- Season with salt.
- Serve an enjoy.

Basil pesto salad dressing

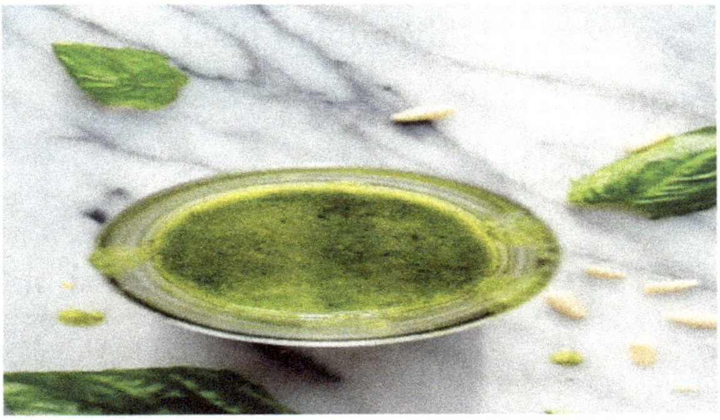

Ingredients

- 4 ounces of chopped romaine lettuce
- ½ cup of fresh basil leaves
- Freshly ground pepper
- 4 ounces of fresh spring greens
- 1 clove garlic

- ¼ teaspoon of salt
- 3 tablespoons of raw pine nuts
- Basil pesto dressing
- ½ cup of extra virgin olive oil
- 2 tablespoons of lemon juice

Directions

- Combine the basil, garlic, and pine nuts in a food blender bowl.
- Pulse until coarsely chopped.
- Drizzle in the olive oil, lemon juice, and salt as the machine is running.
- Season with freshly ground black pepper and blend until smooth.
- Serve and enjoy.

Simple beet arugula and feta salad with balsamic thyme dressing

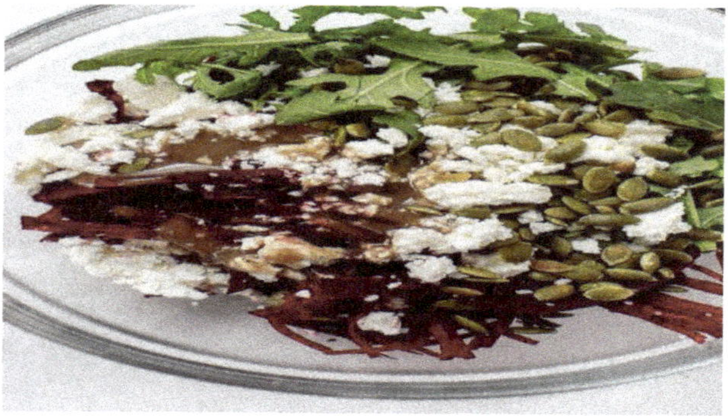

Ingredients

- ¼ cup of crumbled feta
- 2 tablespoons of pepitas
- Balsamic thyme dressing
- 2 medium red beets
- Handful of arugula, roughly chopped

Directions

- Toast the pepitas over a medium heat until fragrant.
- Transfer to a bowl to cool.
- Prepare and stack the rounds of beets on top of each other and slice them into long, thin matchsticks.
- In a medium-sized serving bowl, combine the beets together with the arugula, crumbled feta, and pepitas.
- Drizzle in enough dressing to coat the salad once tossed.
- Serve and enjoy.

Ginger salad dressing

The ginger salad dressing has a striking flavor drawn from the ginger balanced with sweetness infused with the maple syrup making it a tasty Mediterranean Sea diet recipe.

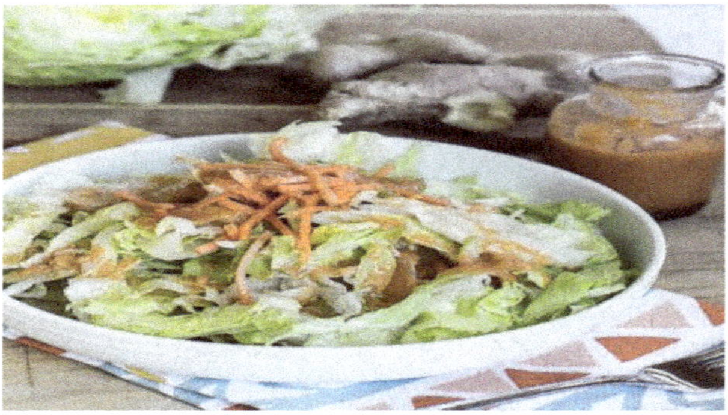

Ingredients

- ½ cup extra-virgin olive oil
- 2 teaspoons of finely grated fresh ginger
- ½ teaspoon of fine sea salt
- 2 tablespoons of apple cider vinegar
- 20 twists of freshly ground black pepper
- 2 tablespoons of Dijon mustard
- 1 tablespoon of maple syrup

Directions

- In a small mixing bowl, whisk all of the ingredients listed until completely blended.
- Taste the seasoning, and adjust accordingly.
- Serve and enjoy.
- Any leftovers can be kept refrigerated until consumed.

Fresh mint dressing

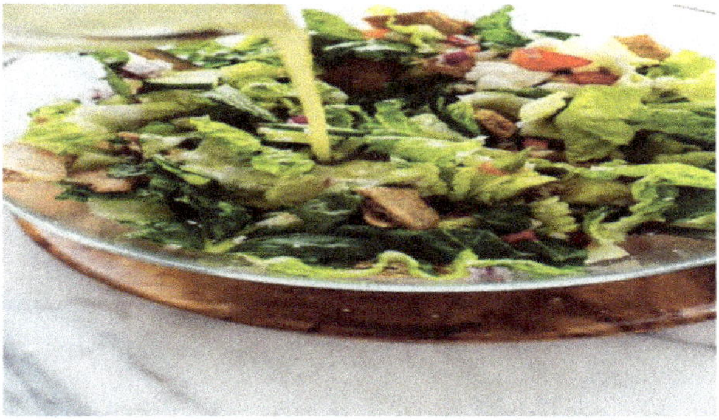

Ingredients

- 2 cloves garlic, roughly chopped
- ½ cup of extra virgin olive oil
- ¼ teaspoon of sea salt
- ½ cup of lemon juice
- ¼ cup of packed fresh mint leaves
- 10 twists of freshly ground black pepper
- 3 tablespoons of honey
- 1 tablespoon of Dijon mustard

Directions

- In a food processor, combine all of the above ingredients and blend until smooth.
- Taste, and adjust the seasoning accordingly.
- Serve and enjoy.
- Any leftover should be refrigerated for up to 1 week.

Conclusion

The Mediterranean Sea diet is not a new type of diet or recipes but rather it emerged several decades ago within the Mediterranean basin. Ultimately, the Mediterranean Sea diet encourages the consumption of natural foods, mainly greens, vegetables, seeds, fruits, nuts, legumes, seafood, whole grains, poultry, and herbs. Consumption of red or lean meat, high sugar and fat content foods are highly discouraged along with the consumption of alcoholic beverages with the exception of few wines. More so, there are various recipes or ways through which one can choose to prepare the Mediterranean Sea diet depending on their taste and preference. The recipes range from vegetable recipes to whole gran meal recipes.

Notably, the Mediterranean Sea diet has exploded to the whole, world due to the tremendous health benefits associated to the consumption of the Mediterranean Sea diet. There seem to be no adverse side effect associated or linked to the consumption of the Mediterranean Sea diet. As such, the population living in the Mediterranean basin that follow the Mediterranean dietary pattern seem to have minimal chances of developing chronic illnesses especially cardiovascular illness, cancer, sickle cell, diabetes, and hypertension among others. In comparison to other healthy diet plans especially the dietary approaches to stop hypertension.

CPSIA information can be obtained
at www.ICGtesting.com
Printed in the USA
BVHW011008200421
605144BV00026B/220

9 781802 661378